Imaging of Athletic Injuries of the Upper Extremity

Editor

MARTIN L. LAZARUS

RADIOLOGIC CLINICS OF NORTH AMERICA

www.radiologic.theclinics.com

Consulting Editor
FRANK H. MILLER

March 2013 • Volume 51 • Number 2

ELSEVIER

1600 John F. Kennedy Boulevard • Suite 1800 • Philadelphia, Pennsylvania, 19103-2899

http://www.theclinics.com

RADIOLOGIC CLINICS OF NORTH AMERICA Volume 51, Number 2
March 2013 ISSN 0033-8389, ISBN 13: 978-1-4557-4888-4

Editor: Adrianne Brigido

Radiologic Clinics of North America (ISSN 0033-8389) is published bimonthly by Elsevier Inc., 360 Park Avenue South, New York, NY 10010-1710. Months of issue are January, March, May, July, September, and November. Periodicals postage paid at New York, NY and additional mailing offices. Subscription prices are USD 438 per year for US individuals, USD 685 per year for US institutions, USD 210 per year for US students and residents, USD 511 per year for Canadian individuals, USD 858 per year for Canadian institutions, USD 630 per year for international individuals, USD 858 per year for international institutions, and USD 302 per year for Canadian and foreign students/residents. To receive student and resident rate, orders must be accompanied by name of affiliated institution, date of term and the signature of program/residency coordinatior on institution letterhead. Orders will be billed at individual rate until proof of status is received. Foreign air speed delivery is included in all *Clinics* subscription prices. All prices are subject to change without notice. **POSTMASTER:** Send address changes to *Radiologic Clinics of North America*, Elsevier Health Sciences Division, Subscription Customer Service, 3251 Riverport Lane, Maryland Heights, MO63043. **Customer Service: Telephone: 1-800-654-2452** (U.S. and Canada); **1-314-447-8871** (outside U.S. and Canada). **Fax: 1-314-447-8029. E-mail: journalscustomerservice-usa@elsevier.com** (for print support); **journalsonlinesupport-usa@elsevier.com** (for online support).

Reprints. For copies of 100 or more of articles in this publication, please contact the Commercial Reprints Department, Elsevier Inc., 360 Park Avenue South, New York, New York 10010-1710. Tel.: (+1) 212-633-3812; Fax: (+1) 212-462-1935; E-mail: reprints@elsevier.com.

Radiologic Clinics of North America also published in Greek Paschalidis Medical Publications, Athens, Greece.

Radiologic Clinics of North America is covered in *MEDLINE/PubMed (Index Medicus), EMBASE/Excerpta Medica, Current Contents/Life Sciences, Current Contents/Clinical Medicine, RSNA Index to Imaging Literature, BIOSIS, Science Citation Index,* and *ISI/BIOMED.*

Printed in the United States of America.

Contributors

CONSULTING EDITOR

FRANK H. MILLER, MD
Professor of Radiology; Chief, Body Imaging
Section and Fellowship Program and GI
Radiology; Medical Director MRI, Department
of Radiology, Feinberg School of Medicine,
Northwestern University, Chicago, Illinois

EDITOR

MARTIN L. LAZARUS, MD
Vice Chairman of Academic Affairs and
Section Chief, Department of Radiology,
Musculoskeletal Imaging, Evanston Hospital,
NorthShore University HealthSystem,
Evanston, Illinois; Clinical Associate Professor
of Radiology, The University of Chicago,
Pritzker School of Medicine, Chicago, Illinois

AUTHORS

JOHN ANNES, MD
Radiology Resident, Department of Radiology,
Stritch School of Medicine, Loyola University
Medical Center, Maywood, Illinois

LAURA W. BANCROFT, MD
Adjunct Professor, University of Central Florida
College of Medicine, Orlando, Florida; Clinical
Professor, Florida State University College of
Medicine, Tallahassee, Florida; Chief of
Musculoskeletal Imaging and Radiology
Specialists of Florida, Department of
Radiology, Florida Hospital, Orlando, Florida

JACOB BOSLEY, MD
Section of Orthopaedic Surgery and
Rehabilitation, Department of Surgery,
The University of Chicago Medical Center,
Chicago, Illinois

TERESA CAPPELLO, MD
Assistant Professor, Department of
Orthopaedic Surgery and Rehabilitation,
Stritch School of Medicine, Loyola University
Medical Center, Maywood, Illinois

HAEMI CHOI, MD
Assistant Professor, Department of Family
Medicine, Loyola University Medical Center,
Maywood, Illinois

NEERU JAYANTHI, MD
Associate Professor, Departments of Family
Medicine, Orthopedic Surgery and
Rehabilitation, Loyola University Medical
Center, Maywood, Illinois

MARTIN L. LAZARUS, MD
Vice Chairman of Academic Affairs and
Section Chief, Department of Radiology,
Musculoskeletal Imaging, Evanston Hospital,
NorthShore University HealthSystem,
Evanston, Illinois; Clinical Associate Professor
of Radiology, The University of Chicago,
Pritzker School of Medicine, Chicago, Illinois

JENNIFER E. LIM-DUNHAM, MD
Associate Professor, Department of Radiology,
Stritch School of Medicine, Loyola University
Medical Center, Maywood, Illinois

LAURIE M. LOMASNEY, MD
Professor, Department of Radiology, Stritch School of Medicine, Loyola University Medical Center, Maywood, Illinois

NEEL B. PATEL, MD
Department of Radiology, The University of Chicago Medical Center, Chicago, Illinois

TIMOTHY G. SANDERS, MD
National Musculoskeletal Imaging (NMSI), Deerfield Beach, Florida

GREGORY SCOTT STACY, MD
Department of Radiology, The University of Chicago Medical Center, Chicago, Illinois

NARAYAN SUNDARAM, MD, MBA
Department of Radiology, The University of Chicago Medical Center, Chicago, Illinois

STEPHEN THOMAS, MD
Department of Radiology, University of Chicago Medical Center, Chicago, Illinois

DANIEL R. WENZKE, MD
Department of Radiology, Evanston Hospital, NorthShore University Health System, Evanston, Illinois; Clinical Assistant Professor, Pritzker School of Medicine, University of Chicago, Chicago, Illinois

MICHAEL B. ZLATKIN, MD
National Musculoskeletal Imaging (NMSI), Deerfield Beach, Florida; Voluntary Professor, School of Medicine, University of Miami, Miami, Florida

Contents

This article summarizes key MR imaging findings in common athletic elbow injuries including little leaguer's elbow, Panner disease, osteochondritis dissecans, olecranon stress fracture, occult fracture, degenerative osteophyte formation, flexor-pronator strain, ulnar collateral ligament tear, lateral ulnar collateral ligament and radial collateral ligament tear, lateral epicondylitis, medial epicondylitis, biceps tear, bicipitoradial bursitis, triceps tear, olecranon bursitis, ulnar neuropathy, posterior interosseous nerve syndrome, and radial tunnel syndrome. The article also summarizes important technical considerations in elbow MR imaging that enhance image quality and contribute to the radiologist's success.

This article highlights the unique patterns of sports-related injury of the upper extremity that radiologists are likely to encounter in children and adolescents. The injuries are classified as acute "use" injuries or chronic "overuse" injuries, and reviewed separately for the shoulder, elbow, and wrist. Recommendations for imaging strategies are provided and characteristic imaging findings are discussed and illustrated.

Although magnetic resonance arthrography is not indicated for every clinical scenario, capsular distention can significantly improve visualization of intra-articular pathologic conditions. With attention to technique, intraarticular injection can be completed successfully with little patient discomfort. This article provides details of the technique for injection of the shoulder, the elbow, and the wrist for optimization of magnetic resonance imaging.

Athletic injuries to the hand are common and encompass a diverse spectrum of injuries. These injuries can include fractures, soft tissue injuries, or both. Athletic injuries to the hand can be due to a variety of mechanisms and can be seen with a variety of sports. Prompt attention and accurate diagnosis should be provided to patients with athletic injuries to the hand to allow for appropriate treatment and to prevent serious complications that may preclude further athletic activity. This article discusses the radiographic evaluation of hand fractures seen in athletes and presents brief descriptions of the clinical management of these injuries.

PROGRAM OBJECTIVE:

The objective of the *Radiologic Clinics of North America* is to keep practicing radiologists and radiology residents up to date with current clinical practice in radiology by providing timely articles reviewing the state of the art in patient care.

TARGET AUDIENCE

Practicing radiologists, radiology residents, and other health care professionals who provide patient care utilizing radiologic findings.

LEARNING OBJECTIVES

Upon completion of this activity, participants will be able to:
1. Discuss conventional radiographic evaluation of athletic injuries to the hand.
2. Compare wrist injuries between high-and-low impact sports.
3. Describe football injuries and throwing injuries of the upper extremities.

ACCREDITATION

The Elsevier Office of Continuing Medical Education (EOCME) is accredited by the Accreditation Council for Continuing Medical Education (ACCME) to provide continuing medical education for physicians.

The EOCME designates this journal-based CME activity for a maximum of 8 *AMA PRA Category 1 Credit*(s)™. Physicians should claim only the credit commensurate with the extent of their participation in the activity.

All other health care professionals completing continuing education credit for this activity will be issued a certificate of participation.

DISCLOSURE OF CONFLICTS OF INTEREST

The EOCME assesses conflict of interest with its instructors, faculty, planners, and other individuals who are in a position to control the content of CME activities. All relevant conflicts of interest that are identified are thoroughly vetted by EOCME for fair balance, scientific objectivity, and patient care recommendations. EOCME is committed to providing its learners with CME activities that promote improvements or quality in healthcare and not a specific proprietary business or a commercial interest.

The planning committee, staff, authors and editors listed below have identified no financial relationships or relationships to products or devices they or their spouse/life partner have with commercial interest related to the content of this CME activity:

John Annes, MD; Laura W. Bancroft, MD; Jacob Bosley, MD; Adrianne Brigido; Teresa Cappello, MD; Haemi Choi, MD; Nicole Congleton; Sandy Lavery; Martin L. Lazarus, MD; Jennifer E. Lim-Dunham, MD; Laurie M. Lomasney, MD; Jill McNair; Frank H. Miller, MD; Karthikeyan Subramaniam; Neel B. Patel, MD; Timothy G. Sanders, MD; Gregory Scott Stacy, MD; Narayan Sundaram, MD, MBA; Stephen Thomas, MD; Daniel R. Wenzke, MD; and Michael B. Zlatkin, MD.

The planning committee, staff, authors and editors listed below have identified financial relationships or relationships to products or devices they or their spouse/life partner have with commercial interest related to the content of this CME activity:

Neeru Jayanthi, MD has received a research grant from American Medical Society for Sports Medicine Foundation; royalties or patents for Epicondyliltis; received Speaker's honorarium at Children's Memorial Hospital, Institute for Sports Medicine Visiting Professor; and received lodging/travel expenses for serving on American Medical Society for Sports Medicine Board of Directors.

UNAPPROVED/OFF-LABEL USE DISCLOSURE

The EOCME requires CME faculty to disclose to the participants:
1. When products or procedures being discussed are off-label, unlabelled, experimental, and/or investigational (not US Food and Drug Administration (FDA) approved); and
2. Any limitations on the information presented, such as data that are preliminary or that represent on-going research, interim analyses, and/or unsupported opinions. Faculty may discuss information about pharmaceutical agents that is outside of FDA-approved labelling. This information is intended solely for CME and is not intended to promote off-label use of these medications. If you have any questions, contact the medical affairs department of the manufacturer for the most recent prescribing information.

TO ENROLL

To enroll in the *Radiologic Clinics of North America* Continuing Medical Education program, call customer service at 1-800-654-2452 or sign up online at http://www.theclinics.com/home/cme. The CME program is available to subscribers for an additional annual fee of USD 288.

METHOD OF PARTICIPATION

In order to claim credit, participants must complete the following:
1. Complete enrolment as indicated above.
2. Read the activity.
3. Complete the CME Test and Evaluation. Participants must achieve a score of 70% on the test. All CME Tests and Evaluations must be completed online.

CME INQUIRIES/SPECIAL NEEDS

For all CME inquiries or special needs, please contact elsevierCME@elsevier.com.

RADIOLOGIC CLINICS OF NORTH AMERICA

Preface

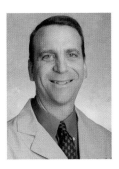

Martin L. Lazarus, MD
Editor

America is a sports-oriented culture. There has been a veritable explosion of active participation in athletics over the last 20 years. This includes people of all age groups. With the advent of Title IX in 1972, women have been involved in sports in increasing numbers, as never before. The young girls that were the first to benefit from the landmark law are now middle aged. There is a constant influx of new female athletes. There are also increasing intensity and pressure placed on our young athletes, male and female, to perform at a higher level. Children and adolescents are being asked to specialize in a single sport, rather than switch sports seasonally.

The end result of these changes is a large increase in the number of injuries that are being imaged. The general radiologist needs to know the basics regarding how to approach these patients—from indications to protocols. MRI will be discussed prominently, as this is the most commonly employed modality when dealing with athletic injuries to the upper extremity. Other modalities such as plain films, CT, and ultrasound are covered. The most up-to-date imaging techniques are reviewed.

Having grown up a prototypical sports fan, I never imagined that it would become a major part of my professional career. Dealing with sports injuries, whether on the recreational, high school, collegiate, or professional level, is more fun than work. I consider myself fortunate to be involved in a project such as this, and the expert contributing authors are a pleasure to read and learn from. This issue discusses topics that include MRI of the elbow, pediatric throwing injuries, a comparison of high-impact and low-impact sports with respect to wrist injuries, MRI of the labrum, an article covering MR arthrography, plain film evaluation of injuries to the hand, and, finally, American football injuries to the upper extremity. I hope that reading this material is a rewarding endeavor for the general and the MSK radiologist.

Martin L. Lazarus, MD
Department of Radiology, MSK Imaging
Evanston Hospital
Northshore University Health System
2650 Ridge Avenue, Evanston, IL 60201, USA

The University of Chicago
Pritzker School of Medicine
924 East 57th Street, Suite 104
Chicago, IL 60637-5415, USA

E-mail address:
MLazarus@northshore.org

Radiol Clin N Am 51 (2013) ix
http://dx.doi.org/10.1016/j.rcl.2013.01.001
0033-8389/13/$ – see front matter © 2013 Published by Elsevier Inc.

MR Imaging of the Elbow in the Injured Athlete

Daniel R. Wenzke, MD[a,b]

KEYWORDS

- Elbow MR imaging • Ulnar collateral ligament tear • Lateral epicondylitis • Panner disease
- Little leaguer's elbow

KEY POINTS

- Equipment and technique choices greatly impact scan quality.
- Familiarity with normal anatomic features helps avoid diagnostic errors.
- Competitive throwing subjects the elbow to chronic valgus stress. This repetitive stress leads to traction injuries medially and compression injuries laterally. Common injury patterns vary based on the degree of skeletal maturity.
- Ulnar collateral ligament (UCL) tear can be a devastating injury to the throwing athlete.
- Medial and lateral epicondylitis are chronic overuse injuries affecting tendons at the elbow. Treatment is usually conservative.
- MRI is very helpful for establishing less common diagnoses such as occult fracture, nerve entrapment, bursitis, and tendon rupture.

INTRODUCTION

MR imaging plays a critical role in evaluating elbow pain in the athlete. Chronic valgus extension loading at the elbow, especially with overhead throwing, causes high compressive forces at the lateral elbow and high tensile (traction) forces at the medial elbow. These high compressive-tensile loads can lead to osseous or chondral injuries (medial epicondyle apophysitis, Panner disease, osteochondritis dissecans [OCD]); olecranon stress fracture; degenerative osteophyte formation; flexor-pronator strain; ulnar collateral ligament (UCL) tear; and ulnar neuropathy. Chronic overuse injury patterns at the elbow are common in racquet sports and include lateral and medial epicondylitis. Athletes in high-energy contact sports, such as American football, weightlifters, or those who abuse anabolic steroids have an increased incidence of distal biceps rupture

and triceps rupture. Finally, nerve entrapment syndromes at the elbow may lead to chronic pain and disability.

This article reviews MR imaging findings of the most common elbow injuries in the athlete. It also summarizes important technical considerations in elbow MR imaging that enhance image quality and contribute to the radiologist's success.

TECHNICAL CONSIDERATIONS
Patient Positioning for Scanning with a Whole-Body MR Imaging System

Optimizing MR imaging of the elbow poses special challenges. The first involves patient positioning. To achieve the best image quality, the body part being scanned should be placed as close to the isocenter of the magnet as possible. When scanning the elbow, this means having the patient lie

No disclosures.
[a] Department of Radiology, Evanston Hospital, NorthShore University HealthSystem, 2650 Ridge Avenue, Evanston, IL 60201, USA; [b] University of Chicago, Pritzker School of Medicine, 924 East 57th Street, Suite 104, Chicago, IL 60637-5415, USA
E-mail address: dwenzke@northshore.org

prone with the arm raised over the head and the elbow in full extension (**Fig. 1**). This is the so-called "superman position." The forearm is placed in supination (ie, thumb up). Patient comfort is critical to reducing motion artifacts. Pillows under the axilla can reduce strain on the shoulder. The arm and hand should be padded for comfort and immobilization.

The superman position has two distinct advantages. The first is improved signal-to-noise from more central positioning in the bore. The second is a wider selection of usable coils. The best coils in modern systems have eight or more receiver channels and parallel imaging capabilities. These features result in marked improvement over older devices. In general, the best available knee coil (eg, eight or more receiver channels) provides the best technical performance in elbow MR imaging when scanning in the superman position.

Unfortunately, many patients cannot tolerate the superman position long enough to complete the study, particularly those with shoulder pain or injury. Some authors have advocated avoiding it altogether for reasons of patient comfort and associated motion artifacts.[1] Although the use of pillows and pads for comfort and immobilization may improve compliance, the radiologist requires a backup strategy.

Patients tolerate supine positioning much more easily. The arm is adducted with the elbow in full extension. The thumb is pointed up (ie, neutral or mild supination at the elbow). The elbow should be as far from the edge of the bore as possible (**Fig. 2**).

Despite substantial advantages in patient comfort, there are three major disadvantages to the

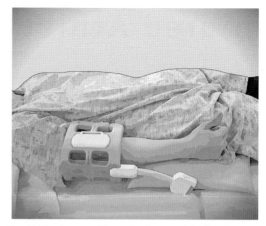

Fig. 2. Supine position. Supine positioning is more comfortable and less likely to result in motion artifact. Disadvantages include reduced signal-to-noise from off-center positioning in the bore and the need to use flex coils. Conventional fat suppression techniques may be compromised by off-center positioning.

supine position. The first is reduced signal-to-noise from the imaging volume location at the periphery of the bore. The second is compromise of frequency-selective fat suppression (FS) techniques (ie, "fat sat") when the elbow is near the edge of the bore (**Fig. 3**). The technologist may

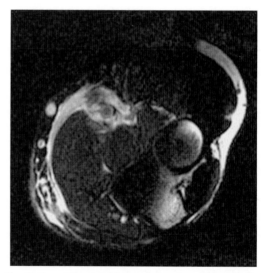

Fig. 3. Poor FS caused by peripheral positioning. The patient is supine with his elbow along his side. Because the elbow is near the edge of the bore, frequency selective FS ("fat sat") fails in the lateral half of the image on this axial T2 FS sequence. If the elbow cannot be placed closer to the center of the bore, short tau inversion recovery (STIR) should be substituted for the T2 or proton density FS sequences. STIR has lower spatial resolution and a longer acquisition time.

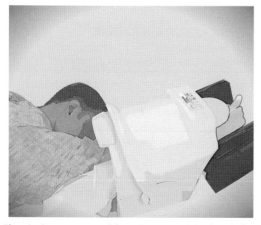

Fig. 1. Superman position. Prone positioning is less comfortable for the patient but offers superior image quality related to isocentric positioning of the elbow in the magnet and superior coil selection. In this case, a high-resolution knee coil is used to image the elbow.

need to convert T2- and proton density (PD)–weighted sequences to short tau inversion recovery sequences (STIR) to achieve homogeneous suppression of the fat signal. The downsides of STIR include lower spatial resolution and longer scan times.

Finally, supine positioning has a large disadvantage in coil selection. The best coils are rigid array coils, such as the knee coils described previously. Unfortunately, these coil devices are cumbersome and usually too large to fit alongside a supine patient. Instead, the technologist must resort to general purpose flexible coils. Although smaller and generally more comfortable, these "flex" coils have an inferior technical profile relative to the best rigid coil systems. Lesser technical performance translates into lower-quality images or longer examination times. More commonly, it results in both.

A third specialized position, termed the flexion, abduction, and supination (FABS) position, enhances visualization of the distal biceps tendon when injury to that structure is the primary clinical concern (**Fig. 4**).[2] The patient lays prone in the scanner with the arm over the head. The elbow is flexed 90 degrees and the thumb is pointed up. This position has patient comfort drawbacks similar to the superman position. Although the elbow is near the isocenter of the magnet, flexion at the joint limits coil selection.

Extremity MR Imaging Systems

Extremity MR imaging systems cost significantly less than whole-body systems and have patient comfort advantages because of an open design. Historically, these types of systems had low-field

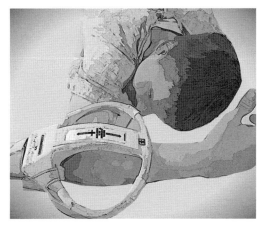

Fig. 4. Flexion, abduction, and supination position. Specialized positioning with the elbow in flexion, abduction, and supination allows enhanced visualization of the distal biceps tendon when evaluation of that structure is the primary concern of the referring clinician.

strength permanent magnets. They suffered from poor signal-to-noise, long scan times, poor spatial resolution, and an inability to obtain thin slices.[3–5] In addition, frequency-selective FS (ie, fat sat) cannot be performed at low-field strength and STIR must be substituted.

The latest generation of extremity MR imaging systems comes with major improvements. The patient rests in a chair and places his or her extremity into a small circular bore. The newer designs include superconducting magnets with field strengths to 1.5 T and the ability to use traditional FS techniques. Image quality improvements are considerable. Unlike whole-body systems where isocentric positioning of the extremity is challenging, extremity MR imaging systems are designed to always have the patient's arm or leg centrally positioned in the magnetic field. Disadvantages relative to traditional whole-body scanners include reduced longitudinal field of view (FOV) coverage and longer scan times compared with the best whole-body systems and coils. Also, the small bore design precludes scanning of the shoulder or hip. Although these dedicated extremity systems may not outperform the best whole-body systems in terms of image quality, the major technical improvements combined with the lower price point and patient comfort advantages may make these scanners viable options for some practices and institutions.

Selecting the MR Imaging Planes

The second challenge is selection of the imaging planes by the MR imaging technologist. In general, MR imaging planes in musculoskeletal radiology use a joint space or joint surface as a landmark to dictate axial, coronal, and sagittal planes. In the elbow, the typical human has a valgus carrying angle of approximately 18 degrees.[6] Therefore, the humerus is not in the same planes as the radius or ulna. In a common approach, the axial plane bisects the humeral epicondyles on a coronal localizer and is perpendicular to the long axis of the humerus on a sagittal localizer.

The coronal plane is more challenging. It bisects the humeral epicondyles on the axial localizer (**Fig. 5A**). On the sagittal localizer, it may be oriented to the humerus, the proximal radius, or with some angle relative to either structure. The goal is to optimize visualization of the anterior band of the UCL. An approach advocated in the literature[7] is to orient the coronal plane to the humerus with 0 to 20 degrees of posterior angulation relative to the long axis of the humerus. If the elbow is fully extended (0 degrees of flexion), a higher degree of posterior angulation (ie, 20 degrees) is used (see **Fig. 5B**). If the elbow is

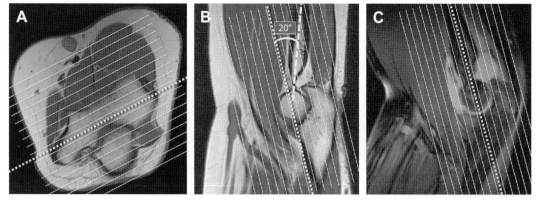

Fig. 5. Coronal plane. (*A*) Coronal plane prescribed on an axial localizer image. The coronal plane bisects the humeral epicondyles on an axial image. (*B*) To optimize visualization of the ulnar collateral ligament, the coronal plane should be angled posteriorly approximately 20 degrees when the elbow is fully extended. (*C*) When the elbow is partially flexed (20 degrees of flexion), the coronal plane is in line with the humeral shaft.

partially flexed (eg, 20 degrees of flexion), the coronal plane is along the humeral axis with 0 degrees of angulation (see **Fig. 5**C).

The sagittal plane is perpendicular to the coronal and axial planes on the axial and coronal localizers, respectively (**Fig. 6**). Coronal and sagittal slices should cover all of the bones. Axial images should include just beyond the radial tuberosity distally to ensure coverage of the distal biceps insertion.

The goal of any imaging protocol is efficient acquisition of high-quality diagnostic images. Although radiologists may tailor elbow protocols to the specific problem being investigated, I prefer to use a single standard protocol for routine imaging and a second protocol for MR arthrography. Although knowledge of specialized

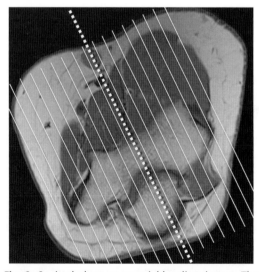

Fig. 6. Sagittal plane on an axial localizer image. The sagittal plane is perpendicular to the coronal plane that bisects the humeral epicondyles.

techniques can occasionally assist in tough cases, "keeping it simple" has many advantages. Simplicity facilitates workflow; improves technologist compliance; and decreases confusion (and therefore the number of telephone calls to the radiologist). I use the superman position and a high-quality knee coil (eight channel or better) whenever possible. Most of the MR imaging systems are 1.5 T with common parameters listed below. Fluid-sensitive sequence options include PD, T2, and STIR. PD with FS (using a longer echo time [TE] of 35–50 milliseconds) has become the preferred sequence in many orthopedic settings, providing a good blend of high signal and fluid sensitivity. STIR sequences can be used when off-center positioning compromises conventional FS.

Standard protocol (all sequences are fast spin echo [FSE]/turbo spin echo [TSE])

> Axial T2 or PD with FS
> Axial T1 or PD
> Coronal T1
> Coronal PD with FS
> Sagittal PD with FS
> Sagittal T1

Arthrogram protocol

> Axial T1 with FS
> Axial T2 or PD with FS
> Axial T1
> Coronal T1 with FS
> Coronal PD with FS
> Sagittal PD with FS
> Sagittal T1 with FS

FOV is typically 12 to 14 cm for all pulse sequences but can be expanded to include

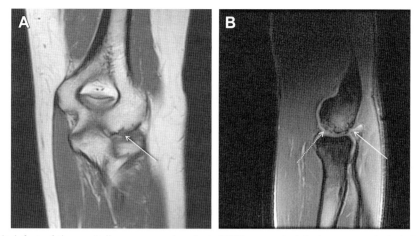

Fig. 7. Pseudodefect of the capitellum, a normal variant. (*A*) The pseudodefect occurs posteriorly in the capitellum (*arrow*). (*B*) In a second patient, the posterior pseudodefect (*solid arrow*) contrasts with the location of pathologic osteochondritis dissecans, which almost always occurs anteriorly on the capitellum (*dotted arrow*).

retracted biceps or triceps tendons. My preferred imaging matrix is 256 × 256 or better. American College of Radiology accreditation requirements for performance of elbow MR imaging[8] include total examination time less than or equal to 45 minutes; slice thickness of less than or equal to 4 mm with an interslice gap of less than or equal to 1.2 mm for axial images; slice thickness of less than or equal to 3 mm with an interslice gap of less than or equal to 1 mm for sagittal and coronal images; and pixel size of less than or equal to 0.6 mm x less than or equal to 0.6 mm for all imaging planes. In practice, this means a 256 × 256 matrix can accommodate up to a 15-cm FOV. A higher resolution matrix can be used with a larger FOV or a lower resolution matrix with a smaller FOV and still meet requirements.

IMPORTANT ANATOMIC FEATURES THAT MAY SIMULATE DISEASE

Radiologists should be familiar with anatomic features at the elbow that may simulate disease. In the posterior aspect of the capitellum, most people have a small depression in the bone. This is referred to as the "pseudodefect of the capitellum" (**Fig. 7**) and should not be mistaken for an osteochondral lesion. True osteochondral lesions tend to occur anteriorly, not posteriorly.[9] Although posterior capitellum impaction injuries may occur, they are uncommon. When present, these injuries are typically associated with additional evidence of injury, such as marrow edema.[10]

Along the trochlea groove of the ulna, many people have a small ridge of bone referred to as the "trochlear ridge" (**Fig. 8A**). It is often irregular

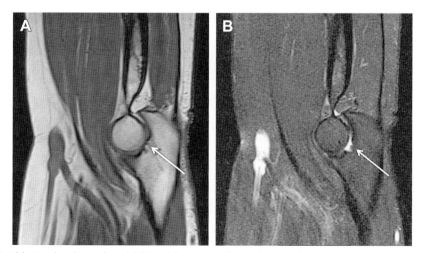

Fig. 8. (*A*) Trochlear ridge (*arrow*) and (*B*) trochlear notch (*arrow*), normal variants.

and not covered by cartilage. This should not be mistaken for an osteophyte or a healed fracture site. At the medial and lateral margins of the ridge, sagittal images may demonstrate small cortical depressions or notches (see **Fig. 8B**).[11]

Finally, synovial plica are often visible in the asymptomatic elbow. The posterolateral plica is almost always visible and should not be mistaken for a pathologic process (**Fig. 9**).[12]

INJURY TO CARTILAGE AND BONE

Little leaguer's elbow refers to a medial-sided elbow injury that occurs in skeletally immature baseball pitchers, most commonly 9 to 12 years old. Repeated valgus stress causes traction injury to the apophysis of the medial epicondyle of the humerus.[13] Also known as medial epicondyle apophysitis, patients present with pain that is relieved by rest. Radiographs may show physeal widening. Widening of 3 to 5 mm may prompt surgical intervention.[14] On MR imaging, fluid-sensitive images show edema adjacent to the apophysis (**Fig. 10**) and can evaluate for any associated injury to the UCL.[15] Any widening of the physis should be measured and reported. Current recommendations include limiting pitch types and pitch counts in young athletes to reduce the incidence of this injury.[14]

Panner disease refers to a lateral-sided elbow injury that also occurs in skeletally immature throwers of the same age group as little leaguer's elbow. Repeated valgus stress causes chronic

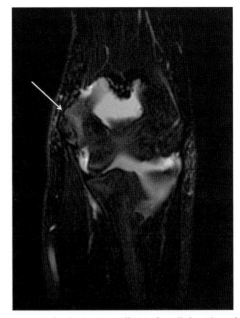

Fig. 10. Little leaguer's elbow (medial epicondyle apophysitis) in a 13-year-old male baseball pitcher. Coronal T2 FS images demonstrate abnormal marrow hyperintensity surrounding the physis of the medial epicondyle of the humerus (*arrow*). The radiologist should measure and report any widening of the physis.

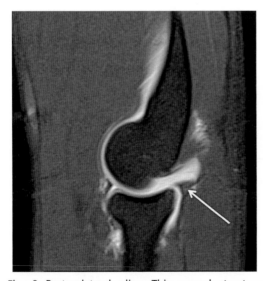

Fig. 9. Posterolateral plica. This normal structure (*arrow*) should not be confused with a loose body or torn ligament.

compression at the lateral elbow, which is thought to compromise the immature blood supply to the unfused capitellar epiphysis. Patients report intermittent pain and stiffness that is relieved by rest and exacerbated by activity.[16,17] Radiographs may show lucency in the capitellum. MR imaging can assist in difficult cases. Fluid-sensitive images show high signal in the marrow surrounding the physis without a chondral defect (**Fig. 11**). In contrast to OCD, the morphology of the bone is preserved. In general, patients do well with conservative therapy.

OCD is also a lateral-sided elbow injury related to chronic compression. It represents a more severe injury on the same spectrum as Panner disease and tends to occur in slightly older throwers, most commonly adolescent male baseball pitchers ages 10 to 16. Patients report diffuse elbow pain and may also have mechanical symptoms, such as catching and locking.[18,19] MR findings include flattening of the subchondral bone and low marrow signal on T1-weighted images. This contrasts with Panner disease, where bone morphology is preserved. The radiologist should report bone fragmentation, chondral defects, and any signs of instability, such as hyperintense fluid signal along the interface between a bone fragment and its base

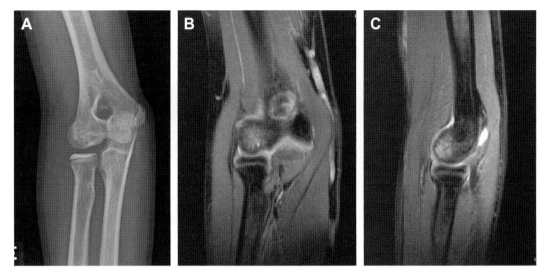

Fig. 11. Panner disease in an 11-year-old female gymnast. (*A*) Plain radiograph of the elbow demonstrates abnormal lucency in the capitellum. Note preservation of the bone contour. Coronal (*B*) and sagittal (*C*) proton density-weighted fat-suppressed images demonstrate abnormal marrow hyperintensity in the capitellum without bone defect or bone deformity. This patient and her twin sister (also a gymnast) had MR imaging examinations on both elbows to evaluate pain. The capitellum had abnormal signal in all four elbows. (*Courtesy of* Alex J. Krasny, MD, Naperville, IL.)

(**Fig. 12**).[20] With MR arthrography, intra-articular contrast extension deep to the fragment implies an unstable lesion.[21] It is important to identify unstable lesions because those patients require surgery. Unfortunately, the sensitivity of MR imaging is imperfect and many patients have unstable lesions at surgery without evidence of instability on preoperative MR imaging.[22,23] Because loose bodies often accompany OCD lesions, the radiologist should inspect the joint space carefully. Although OCD lesions occur in the capitellum in most cases, they may rarely occur at other articular surfaces, such as the humeral trochlea or radial head (**Fig. 13**).[24]

MR imaging can assist in the diagnosis of occult fracture (**Fig. 14**) or with olecranon stress reaction and stress fracture (**Fig. 15**). In the setting of stress reaction, fluid-sensitive MR images demonstrate high signal in the olecranon bone marrow. When stress reaction progresses to fracture, MR imaging shows an irregular T1 hypointense line surrounded by abnormal marrow signal. Olecranon stress

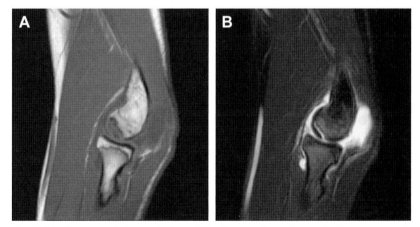

Fig. 12. Osteochondritis dissecans of the capitellum. This 17-year-old male tennis player reported acute onset of sharp pain during a match. (*A*) Sagittal T1-weighted images demonstrate flattening of the cortex of the capitellum and abnormal low T1 signal. (*B*) Sagittal T2-weighted images show hyperintense fluid undercutting the capitellum fragment, diagnostic of an unstable fragment. The treatment is surgical.

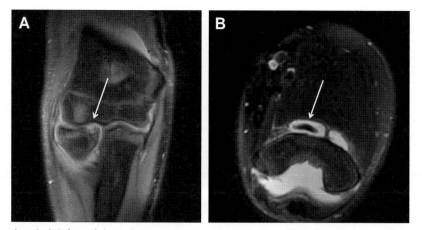

Fig. 13. Osteochondral defect of the radial head in a 14-year-old male baseball pitcher. (*A*) Coronal PD-weighted fat-suppressed images demonstrate an osteochondral defect in the radial head (*arrow*). (*B*) Axial T2-weighted fat-suppressed images show a loose fragment (*arrow*) in the anterior joint space.

injuries are associated with upper limb–dominated sports, such as baseball, tennis, weightlifting, and gymnastics.[25–31]

Olecranon osteophytes (**Fig. 16**) occur postero-medially in the overhead thrower with chronic valgus extension overload.[32] They can cause significant disability and are sometimes resected surgically. Olecranon osteophytes may occur posterolaterally with repeated hyperextension injury, a pattern dubbed boxer's elbow. During missed punches, boxers hyperextend at the elbow without valgus strain.[33] In handball goalie's elbow,

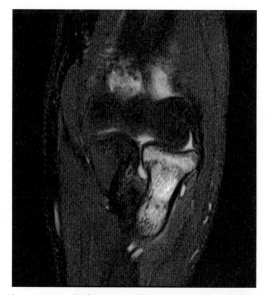

Fig. 14. Occult fracture of the proximal radius in a 16-year-old boy. Initial radiographs did not show a fracture. Coronal T2 fat-suppressed MR clearly demonstrates abnormal signal and a hypointense fracture line in the proximal radius.

repetitive hyperextension during shot-blocking can lead to osteophyte formation or to painful inflam-mation of the posterolateral synovial plica.[34,35]

Loose body formation can complicate many of these disorders and may even result from osteo-phyte fracture. Symptoms include catching or locking. Loose bodies can accelerate degenera-tive changes and are often removed surgically. Gradient echo sequences or MR arthrography can improve detection (**Fig. 17**).

INJURY TO LIGAMENTS

In the medial elbow, the UCL (also known as the medial collateral ligament) is the main stabilizer against valgus stress. Rupture of this ligament is a catastrophic injury to the athlete. Baseball players, especially high-velocity pitchers, are particularly susceptible.[36] In women's sports, soft-ball players and gymnasts have an increased inci-dence of UCL tearing.[37] Absence from competition during recovery typically lasts a year or more. Clinical assessment of UCL integrity is often limited, particularly in the setting of partial tears. Therefore, MR imaging plays an important role in the diagnosis.

The UCL consists of three distinct bundles: (1) anterior, (2) posterior, and (3) transverse. The anterior bundle is the most important stabilizer and the one most frequently injured. It originates at the medial epicondyle of the humerus and inserts on the sublime tubercle of the ulna (the medial margin of the coronoid process) approximately 3 to 4 mm distal to the articular surface. MR arthrography is the study of choice to evaluate for UCL injury.

As in the assessment of other ligamentous injuries, the radiologist should look closely for fluid

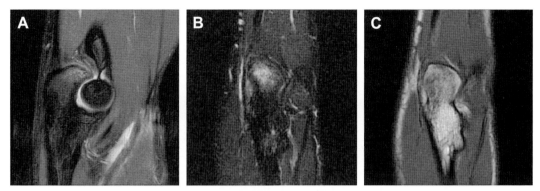

Fig. 15. Olecranon stress reaction in a 16-year-old male baseball pitcher. Sagittal PD (A) and coronal T2 (B) fat-suppressed images show abnormal increased signal in the marrow of the posterior olecranon. (C) A single coronal T1-weighted image shows abnormal low marrow signal. A small irregular hypointense line may represent early stress fracturing.

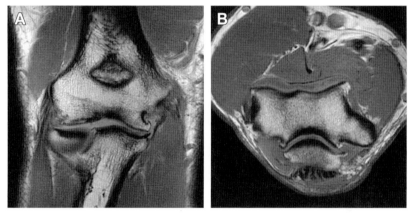

Fig. 16. Olecranon osteophytes. (A, B) In a 32-year-old lineman in the National Football League, osteophytes are present posteromedially and posterolaterally.

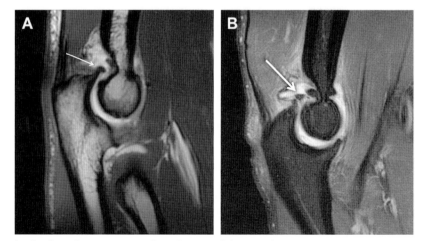

Fig. 17. Loose body after olecranon osteophyte fracture. (A) Sagittal T1 imaging during MR arthrography shows prominent osteophytes at the olecranon (arrow) in the elbow of a 29-year-old lineman in the National Football League. (B) The patient returned several years later with loose body formation thought to have resulted from olecranon osteophyte fracture (arrow).

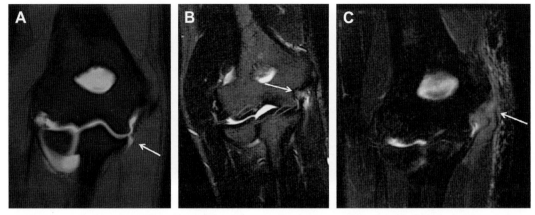

Fig. 18. UCL, complete tears. (*A*) MR arthrography in a 20-year-old college baseball pitcher shows complete tearing of the UCL from its distal attachment on the sublime tubercle of the ulna. Abnormal contrast extension along the medial margin of the sublime tubercle constitutes the "arthrographic T sign" (*arrow*). (*B*) Coronal PD FS imaging shows a mid-substance tear (*arrow*) in a male jujitsu competitor. (*C*) Coronal T2 FS image shows a complete tear of the proximal UCL (*arrow*) in a third patient.

signal in or around the ligament substance, ligamentous laxity or wavy fibers, fiber disruption, and adjacent marrow signal abnormality (**Fig. 18**). The arthrographic T-sign also indicates tearing and is a valuable clue for diagnosing partial thickness tears of the UCL (**Fig. 19**). The sign is present when injected contrast extends distally from the joint line along the cortical margin of the sublime tubercle as seen on coronal images.[38,39] Strict attention to technique in selecting the coronal imaging plane is recommended when evaluating for UCL injury.

Patients that fail conservative therapy with rehabilitation are treated with reconstructive surgery, known as "Tommy John" surgery in reference to the first Major League baseball pitcher to undergo the procedure. Young patients with tears at the proximal or distal end may be candidates for primary repair.[40]

The radial collateral ligament (RCL) complex has four major components at the lateral elbow: (1) the RCL (also known as the lateral collateral ligament); (2) the lateral UCL (LUCL); (3) the annular ligament; and (4) an accessory LUCL. There is wide anatomic variation among individuals.[41] The LUCL extends from the inferior aspect of the lateral humeral epicondyle proximally to the supinator crest of the ulna distally. Typically, the proximal portions of the RCL proper and the LUCL are indistinguishable at dissection.[42,43]

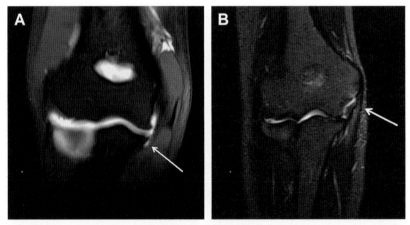

Fig. 19. UCL, partial tears. (*A*) MR arthrography demonstrates the "T sign" of contrast extension along the lateral margin of the sublime tubercle (*arrow*) in a 15-year-old football player with a partial-thickness distal substance tear. (*B*) The UCL has wavy, lax fibers (*arrow*) in this 18-year-old female soccer goalie. The proximal substance is attenuated with mild marrow edema deep to the humeral attachment site. ([*A*] *Courtesy of* Alex J. Krasny, MD, Naperville, IL.)

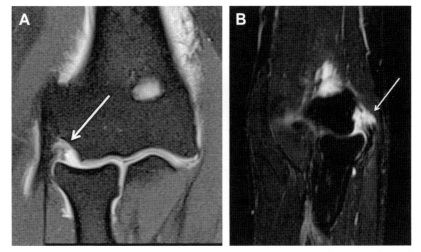

Fig. 20. LUCL tear. (*A*) MR arthrography shows tearing of the proximal portion of the LUCL (*arrow*) in an 18-year-old male baseball pitcher. The immediately adjacent radial collateral ligament (RCL) is intact. (*B*) In a second patient with a more extensive injury, the proximal LUCL and RCL are torn (*arrow*).

LUCL injury is an important entity that can lead to posterolateral rotatory instability of the elbow. During elbow flexion, the radius and ulna abnormally displace into external rotation and valgus. Patients report pain and mechanical symptoms. This entity is difficult to diagnose clinically and often requires assessment of joint laxity while under anesthesia.[44] MR imaging the LUCL can be challenging, especially in the setting of chronic instability.[43,45,46] The LUCL most often tears proximally. Because the RCL and LUCL share a common origin,[43] injury often involves both structures (**Fig. 20**). MR imaging findings may include ligamentous laxity or discontinuity. Sagittal images

Table 1
Characterizing tendon pathology with MR imaging

Pathology	MR Imaging Findings	MR Imaging Report
Degeneration or tendinosis	↑ T1, PD signal Intermediate/low T2 signal Calcification: ↓ signal on all sequences	Mild, moderate, or severe Calcification
Partial tear	↑ T1, PD signal Acute: ↑ T2 signal within or surrounding tendon Chronic: intermediate/low T2 signal (often coexists with degeneration)	Acute or chronic Location: insertion, distance (cm) from insertion, myotendinous junction Tendon caliber: thinned, thickened, or normal % fibers involved in acute tears: <25%, 25%–50%, >50%, and so forth Retraction (cm) of torn fibers Muscle edema or atrophy Marrow edema or fluid collections at tendon attachment sites
Complete tear	Complete disruption of the tendon ↑ T2 signal fluid in a tendon gap	Gap or retraction (cm) of torn fibers Quality of tendon remnants (eg, sharp margins or very frayed or severe degeneration) Muscle edema or atrophy Marrow edema or fluid collections at tendon attachment sites

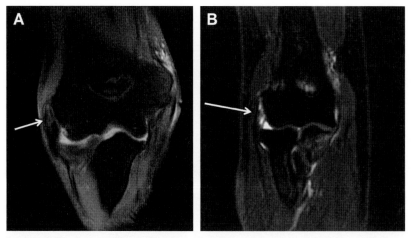

Fig. 21. Lateral epicondylitis (tennis elbow). (*A*) Coronal PD FS imaging shows thickening of the common extensor tendon with intermediate signal (*arrow*), typical of tendinosis. (*B*) In a second patient, hyperintense fluid signal within the common extensor tendon (*arrow*) is diagnostic of partial tearing.

may show posterior subluxation of the radial head relative to the capitellum.[47] There may be bony avulsion at the proximal ligamentous attachment site or underlying marrow edema in the humerus. Treatment options include ligament repair or isometric reconstruction with a tendon graft.[44]

INJURY TO MUSCLES AND TENDONS

Athletes often present with injuries to myotendinous structures from either acute events or from chronic overuse **Table 1**. Lateral epicondylitis is the most common tendon pathology encountered in the elbow. Racquet sport players (tennis, squash, and racquetball) frequently suffer this injury, leading to the name "tennis elbow." A chronic overuse

injury, it results from repetitive microtrauma to the common extensor tendon at the lateral epicondyle during supination, dorsiflexion, and radial deviation. Tearing predominates in the extensor carpi radialis brevis tendon component of the common extensor tendon (**Fig. 21**). With continued chronic stress, larger tears and granulation tissue can develop. Granulation tissue (intermediate signal on fluid-sensitive sequences) should be identified when present because it can cause chronic pain that is treatable with surgical resection.[48]

Medial epicondylitis or golfer's elbow represents injury to the flexor-pronator muscle group at its origin on the medial epicondyle of the humerus. It occurs much less commonly than lateral epicondylitis. Overhead throwers and many

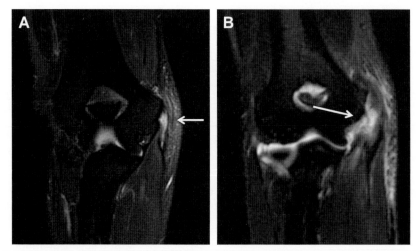

Fig. 22. Medial epicondylitis (golfer's elbow). (*A*) Coronal PD FS imaging shows hyperintense fluid signal in the proximal common flexor tendon (*arrow*), diagnostic of partial tear. (*B*) Imaging in a second patient shows more extensive tearing of the common flexor tendon and the adjacent ulnar collateral ligament (*arrow*).

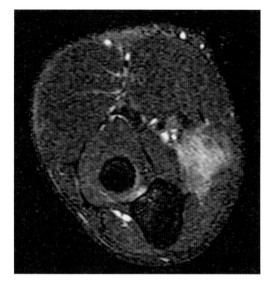

Fig. 23. Flexor-pronator strain in an 18-year-old male wrestler. Axial imaging demonstrates feathery T2 hyper-intense signal in the flexor-pronator muscle group.

other groups of athletes (golf, racquet sports, bowling, and archery) may suffer this injury. The chronic overuse pattern predominantly affects the flexor carpi radialis and pronator teres muscles. Larger tears may involve the whole group (**Fig. 22**).[49] As with lateral epicondylitis, the radiologist should identify tendinosis, tendon tears, calcification, and granulation tissue. In addition to the chronic injury pattern, athletes may present with an acute injury known as "flexor-pronator strain." In these cases, MR imaging demonstrates high signal in the flexor-pronator muscle bellies on fluid-sensitive sequences (**Fig. 23**).

Current therapies for lateral and medial epicondylitis include activity restriction and immobilization. Although corticosteroid injection may improve short-term symptoms, longer-term outcomes are inferior to conservative therapy. Newer therapies have shown encouraging results and include injections of autologous blood or platelet-rich plasma.[50]

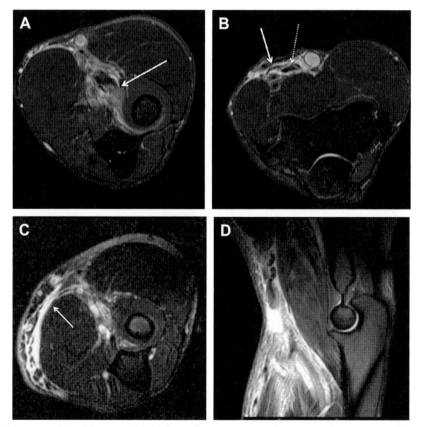

Fig. 24. Distal rupture of the biceps tendon. (*A*) Axial T2 FS imaging shows complete rupture of the distal biceps tendon (*arrow*) from its distal attachment on the radial tuberosity with minimal retraction. There is surrounding T2 hyperintense edema and hemorrhage. (*B*) More proximal imaging shows an intact lacertus fibrosis (*solid arrow*) attaching to the biceps tendon (*dotted arrow*). (*C*) In a second patient, lacertus fibrosis is disrupted (*arrow*) and (*D*) the biceps tendon is retracted proximally into the arm.

Although relatively rare in the young athlete population, distal biceps tendon rupture is a serious injury.[51] In football players, this may occur with forced extension of a flexed elbow while making a tackle. For weightlifters, force generated during the biceps curl may overwhelm the tendon, which tears near its insertion on the radial tuberosity. Patients often report sharp pain and a popping sensation. On physical examination, there is bruising and prominence of the biceps muscle belly, the so-called "Popeye" deformity. Placing the patient in the flexion, abduction, and supination position during MR imaging can improve visualization of distal biceps tears. The radiologist should discriminate between partial- and full-thickness tears; estimate the amount of tendon retraction; and evaluate the integrity of the bicipital aponeurosis (also known as "lacertus fibrosis"). The tendon retracts proximally with complete tears, leaving high signal fluid in the antecubital fossa (**Fig. 24**A). Proximal retraction is more pronounced when there is associated tearing of the bicipital aponeurosis (see **Fig. 24**B). Partial tears may demonstrate fluid signal in the tendon substance or peritendinous edema. Chronic changes of tendinosis (intermediate signal on fluid-sensitive sequences) may coexist with acute tears or represent the only visible tendon pathology.[52–54]

Bicipitoradial bursitis refers to fluid distention of the bicipitoradial bursa. Frequently the result of repetitive mechanical trauma,[55] bursitis may accompany bicipital tendinosis or tearing. The bursa lies posterior to the distal biceps tendon and anterior to the cortex of the radial tuberosity, reducing friction between the two structures during movement. During pronation, the bursa is compressed between the cortex of the radius and the distal biceps tendon. With bursitis, axial MR images demonstrate fluid distention of the bursa (**Fig. 25**), which can restrict the range of motion or exert mass effect on the adjacent radial nerve. If the superficial sensory nerve components of the radial nerve are affected, the patient may present with forearm pain but no motor deficit (see radial tunnel syndrome discussed later). If the deep motor nerve branch (ie, the posterior interosseous nerve) is affected, the patient may present with motor weakness; abnormal nerve conduction by electromyography; and abnormal MR imaging signal in the forearm extensors (see posterior interosseous nerve syndrome discussed later).[56]

Triceps tendon rupture is rare in athletes. Common mechanisms include falling on an outstretched hand, trauma from a direct blow, and forced flexion during active extension.[57] Body

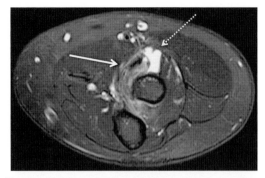

Fig. 25. Bicipitoradial bursitis. Severe biceps tendinosis (*solid arrow*) is accompanied by distention of the bicipitoradial bursa (*dotted arrow*).

builders and athletes involved in violent contact sports, such as professional American football, are at higher risk. The greater prevalence of anabolic steroid use in these populations likely plays a role.[57–59] The radiologist should identify the site of tearing (insertion, myotendinous junction, or intramuscular); discriminate partial from complete tear; and estimate the amount of any tendon retraction.[59,60] Sagittal and axial fluid-sensitive images with FS typically best show the tear. Tears most commonly occur distally at the olecranon insertion and may be accompanied by a small avulsion fracture (**Fig. 26**). Partial tears typically affect the central third of the tendon distally. The normal broad and striated appearance of the distal triceps tendon should not be misinterpreted as pathologic. The FOV may need

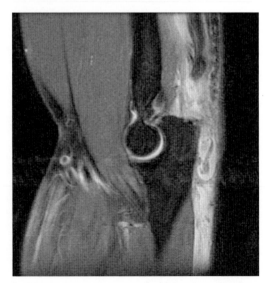

Fig. 26. Triceps rupture. Sagittal T2 FS imaging shows complete rupture of the triceps tendon from its attachment on the olecranon. Edema and hemorrhage extends into the surrounding soft tissue including the olecranon bursa.

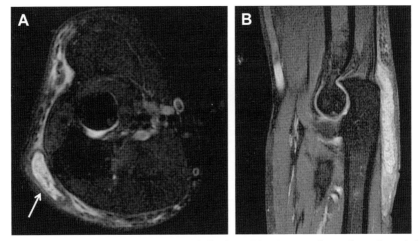

Fig. 27. Olecranon bursitis. Axial (*A*) and sagittal (*B*) fluid-sensitive images show distention of the olecranon bursa (*arrow*). Any visible fluid in the olecranon bursa is abnormal and should be considered bursitis.

to be extended cranially to fully evaluate the degree of tendon retraction.

Olecranon bursitis may occur in isolation or in association with triceps tears. Previous studies have reported an increased incidence in American football players who play on artificial turf.[61] More recently, a series of cases was reported in a group of soldiers involved in intensive infantry training who suffered abrasions to the elbow.[62] Best seen on fluid-sensitive images, the olecranon bursa overlies the olecranon posteriorly. Normally, no hyperintense fluid will be is visible. Any distention with fluid should be considered bursitis (**Fig. 27**). MR imaging may show edema or thickening of the adjacent triceps tendon. Secondary infection can occur even when a break in the skin is not detectable clinically. The MR imaging findings of septic olecranon bursitis overlap with those of noninfected cases. When intravenous contrast is administered, an absence of bursa and soft tissue enhancement makes septic bursitis very unlikely.[63] Because osteomyelitis may occur secondary to septic olecranon bursitis, the radiologist should carefully evaluate the marrow signal of the underlying olecranon.[63]

In climber's elbow, patients present with acute onset of cubital fossa region pain. MR imaging shows tearing of the brachialis muscle in the region of the myotendinous junction proximal to the elbow (**Fig. 28**).[64,65] Overall, acute brachialis muscle tears are rare and usually associated with other injuries.[66]

NERVE ENTRAPMENT OR INJURY

Ulnar neuritis may complicate elbow injuries. For example, tearing of the UCL results in increased traction stresses on the nerve and can lead to neurologic symptoms. Cubital tunnel syndrome refers to the clinical manifestations of ulnar nerve compression, which may occur in the setting of osteophytes, muscle hypertrophy, or an anomalous accessory muscle called the anconeus epitrochlearis.[67] Found in approximately 11% of the population,[68] this muscle arises from the medial border of the olecranon and triceps and inserts on the medial epicondyle of the humerus. It overlies the ulnar nerve in the cubital tunnel and can cause nerve compression (**Fig. 29**).[69,70] With ulnar neuritis, MR imaging findings include high fluid

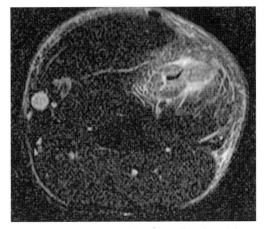

Fig. 28. Brachialis strain (climber's elbow). Axial STIR imaging shows abnormal feathery hyperintensity in the brachialis muscle belly in this patient who suffered an injury while doing pull-ups. Note the poor signal-to-noise of STIR imaging, which was used to improve peripheral fat suppression while scanning in the supine position (see example in **Fig. 3**).

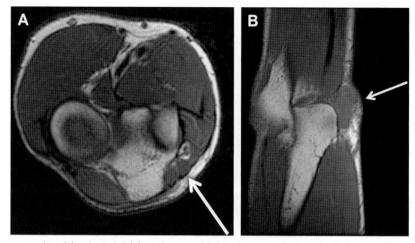

Fig. 29. Anconeus epitrochlearis. Axial (*A*) and coronal (*B*) T1 images of an anomalous accessory muscle (*arrow*) superficial to the ulnar nerve in the cubital tunnel. This muscle can contribute to ulnar compression that results in ulnar neuropathy (ie, cubital tunnel syndrome).

signal in the ulnar nerve at the cubital tunnel (**Fig. 30**).[71,72] Caution is required, however, because a recent study showed high signal in the ulnar nerve in 60% of asymptomatic individuals.[73] Imaging with the elbow in flexion enhances detection of ulnar nerve subluxation, which may be contributory.[74,75] In more severe cases of denervation injury, MR imaging may show edema or fatty atrophy in the muscle bellies of flexor digitorum profundus, flexor carpi ulnaris, or in the intrinsic muscles of the hand. Edema is hyperintense on fluid-sensitive images, whereas atrophy shows bright fat signal replacing the intermediate signal of muscle tissue on T1-weighted images.[71]

Direct visualization of the median and radial nerves at the elbow is typically limited. The radiologist should be familiar with patterns of muscle edema and atrophy that suggest an underlying neuropathy.

Posterior interosseous nerve syndrome is a motor neuropathy related to extrinsic compression. The radial nerve branches at the elbow, giving rise to the posterior interosseous and superficial radial nerves. Compression of the posterior interosseous nerve branch may occur where it plunges into the proximal supinator muscle belly at the elbow. Causes of compression include fibrous bands at the radial head; prominent radial vessels; a distended bicipitoradial bursa; a prominent edge of the extensor carpi radialis brevis; and the proximal edge of the superficial head of the supinator muscle (known as the "arcade of

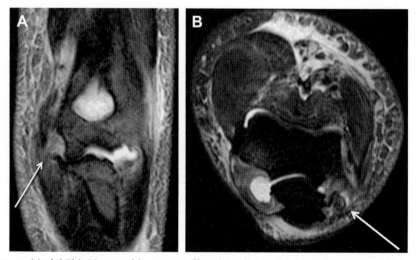

Fig. 30. Ulnar neuritis. (*A*) This 29-year-old woman suffered an ulnar collateral ligament tear (*arrow*) complicated by ulnar neuritis. (*B*) Axial MR imaging shows abnormal thickening and T2 hyperintensity of the ulnar nerve (*arrow*).

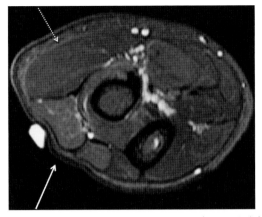

Fig. 31. Posterior interosseous nerve syndrome. Axial T2 FS imaging shows the typical pattern of abnormal high signal in the extensor compartment (*solid arrow*) with sparing of extensor carpi radialis brevis (*dotted arrow*). (*Courtesy of* Alex J. Krasny, MD, Naperville, IL.)

Frohse"). The site of compression may not be detectable with imaging.

On MR imaging, abnormal signal may or may not be visible within the posterior interosseous nerve itself. Rather, the radiologist should suggest the diagnosis after identifying the typical pattern of denervation edema or atrophy in the supinator muscle and extensor muscle group. Fluid-sensitive FS images show diffuse feathery hyperintensity uniformly throughout the affected muscle bellies (see **Fig. 31**). In longstanding cases, this may be accompanied by similarly uniform, diffuse T1 hyperintense fat signal and loss of muscle bulk. These findings indicate chronic denervation atrophy and fatty replacement (T1-weighted without FS). Of note, the extensor carpi radialis longus and brevis

muscles are not innervated by the posterior interosseous nerve and are therefore spared.[71]

Radial tunnel syndrome is a controversial entity described as a sensory neuropathy. It is characterized clinically by lateral forearm pain without motor weakness. Although the posterior interosseous nerve is primarily a motor nerve structure, it carries sensory fibers from the wrist and forearm muscles. In contrast to the motor neuropathy of posterior interosseous nerve syndrome, electromyography studies are typically normal in radial tunnel syndrome. Some authors have suggested that compression may occur more distally along the course of the posterior interosseous nerve in radial tunnel syndrome.[76]

In a minority of cases, MR imaging demonstrates diffuse hyperintense fluid signal in the supinator muscle belly (**Fig. 32**) and rarely in the forearm extensors.[77] This contrasts with the more extensive pattern of involvement seen with posterior interosseous nerve syndrome. The understanding of radial tunnel syndrome continues to evolve.

REFERENCES

1. Potter HG, Schachar J, Jawetz S. Imaging of the elbow. Operat Tech Orthop 2009;19(4):199–208.

2. Giuffre BM, Moss MJ. Optimal positioning for MRI of the distal biceps brachii tendon: flexed abducted supinated view. AJR Am J Roentgenol 2004; 182(4):944–6.

3. Parizel PM, Dijkstra HA, Geenen GP, et al. Low-field versus high-field MR imaging of the knee: a comparison of signal behaviour and diagnostic performance. Eur J Radiol 1995;19(2):132–8.

4. Magee T, Shapiro M, Williams D. Comparison of high-field-strength versus low-field-strength MRI of the shoulder. AJR Am J Roentgenol 2003;181(5):1211–5.

5. Sanal HT, Cardoso F, Chen L, et al. Office-based versus high-field strength MRI: diagnostic and technical considerations. Sports Med Arthrosc 2009; 17(1):31–9.

6. Beals RK. The normal carrying angle of the elbow. A radiographic study of 422 patients. Clin Orthop Relat Res 1976;(119):194–6.

7. Cotten A, Jacobson J, Brossmann J, et al. Collateral ligaments of the elbow: conventional MR imaging and MR arthrography with coronal oblique plane and elbow flexion. Radiology 1997;204(3):806–12.

8. American College of Radiology. MRI Accreditation Program Clinical Image Quality Guide. 2008. Available at: http://www.acr.org/~/media/ACR/Documents/Accreditation/MRI/ClinicalGuide.pdf. Accessed March 7, 2012.

9. Rosenberg ZS, Beltran J, Cheung YY. Pseudodefect of the capitellum: potential MR imaging pitfall. Radiology 1994;191(3):821–3.

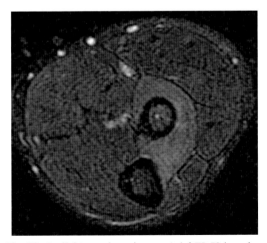

Fig. 32. Radial tunnel syndrome. Axial T2 FS imaging in a 16-year-old boy with forearm pain shows diffuse hyperintensity in the muscle belly of supinator with sparing of the other muscles.

10. Rosenberg ZS, Blutreich SI, Schweitzer ME, et al. MRI features of posterior capitellar impaction injuries. AJR Am J Roentgenol 2008;190(2):435–41.

11. Rosenberg ZS, Beltran J, Cheung Y, et al. MR imaging of the elbow: normal variant and potential diagnostic pitfalls of the trochlear groove and cubital tunnel. AJR Am J Roentgenol 1995;164(2):415–8.

12. Husarik DB, Saupe N, Pfirrmann CW, et al. Ligaments and plicae of the elbow: normal MR imaging variability in 60 asymptomatic subjects. Radiology 2010;257(1):185–94.

13. Klingele KE, Kocher MS. Little league elbow: valgus overload injury in the paediatric athlete. Sports Med 2002;32(15):1005–15.

14. Benjamin HJ, Briner WW Jr. Little league elbow. Clin J Sport Med 2005;15(1):37–40.

15. Hang DW, Chao CM, Hang YS. A clinical and roentgenographic study of little league elbow. Am J Sports Med 2004;32(1):79–84.

16. Wheeless textbook of orthopaedics. United States: s.n.; 1996.

17. Kijowski R, Tuite MJ. Pediatric throwing injuries of the elbow. Semin Musculoskelet Radiol 2010;14(4): 419–29.

18. Nissen CW. Osteochondritis dissecans of the elbow. Conn Med 2010;74(8):453–6.

19. Baker CLIII, Romeo AA, Baker CL Jr. Osteochondritis dissecans of the capitellum. Am J Sports Med 2010;38(9):1917–28.

20. Takahara M, Ogino T, Takagi M, et al. Natural progression of osteochondritis dissecans of the humeral capitellum: initial observations. Radiology 2000;216(1):207–12.

21. Nelson DW, DiPaola J, Colville M, et al. Osteochondritis dissecans of the talus and knee: prospective comparison of MR and arthroscopic classifications. J Comput Assist Tomogr 1990;14(5):804–8.

22. Iwasaki N, Kamishima T, Kato H, et al. A retrospective evaluation of magnetic resonance imaging effectiveness on capitellar osteochondritis dissecans among overhead athletes. Am J Sports Med 2012;40(3):624–30.

23. Heywood CS, Benke MT, Brindle K, et al. Correlation of magnetic resonance imaging to arthroscopic findings of stability in juvenile osteochondritis dissecans. Arthroscopy 2011;27(2):194–9.

24. Marshall KW, Marshall DL, Busch MT, et al. Osteochondral lesions of the humeral trochlea in the young athlete. Skeletal Radiol 2009;38(5):479–91.

25. Nuber GW, Diment MT. Olecranon stress fractures in throwers. A report of two cases and a review of the literature. Clin Orthop Relat Res 1992;(278):58–61.

26. Suzuki K, Minami A, Suenaga N, et al. Oblique stress fracture of the olecranon in baseball pitchers. J Shoulder Elbow Surg 1997;6(5):491–4.

27. Brukner P. Stress fractures of the upper limb. Sports Med 1998;26(6):415–24.

28. Hulkko A, Orava S, Nikula P. Stress fractures of the olecranon in javelin throwers. Int J Sports Med 1986;7(4):210–3.

29. Rao PS, Rao SK, Navadgi BC. Olecranon stress fracture in a weight lifter: a case report. Br J Sports Med 2001;35(1):72–3.

30. Maffulli N, Chan D, Aldridge MJ. Overuse injuries of the olecranon in young gymnasts. J Bone Joint Surg Br 1992;74(2):305–8.

31. Shinozaki T, Kondo T, Takagishi K. Olecranon stress fracture in a young tower-diving swimmer. Orthopedics 2006;29(8):693–4.

32. Wilson FD, Andrews JR, Blackburn TA, et al. Valgus extension overload in the pitching elbow. Am J Sports Med 1983;11(2):83–8.

33. Valkering KP, van der Hoeven H, Pijnenburg BC. Posterolateral elbow impingement in professional boxers. Am J Sports Med 2008;36(2):328–32.

34. Tyrdal S, Finnanger AM. Osseous manifestations of handball goalie's elbow. Scand J Med Sci Sports 1999;9(2):92–7.

35. Popovic N, Lemaire R. Hyperextension trauma to the elbow: radiological and ultrasonographic evaluation in handball goalkeepers. Br J Sports Med 2002; 36(6):452–6.

36. Bushnell BD, Anz AW, Noonan TJ, et al. Association of maximum pitch velocity and elbow injury in professional baseball pitchers. Am J Sports Med 2010;38(4):728–32.

37. Argo D, Trenhaile SW, Savoie FHIII, et al. Operative treatment of ulnar collateral ligament insufficiency of the elbow in female athletes. Am J Sports Med 2006; 34(3):431–7.

38. Timmerman LA, Schwartz ML, Andrews JR. Preoperative evaluation of the ulnar collateral ligament by magnetic resonance imaging and computed tomography arthrography. Evaluation in 25 baseball players with surgical confirmation. Am J Sports Med 1994;22(1):26–31 [discussion: 32].

39. Timmerman LA, Andrews JR. Undersurface tear of the ulnar collateral ligament in baseball players. A newly recognized lesion. Am J Sports Med 1994; 22(1):33–6.

40. Savoie FHIII, Trenhaile SW, Roberts J, et al. Primary repair of ulnar collateral ligament injuries of the elbow in young athletes: a case series of injuries to the proximal and distal ends of the ligament. Am J Sports Med 2008;36(6):1066–72.

41. Morrey BF, An KN. Functional anatomy of the ligaments of the elbow. Clin Orthop Relat Res 1985;(201):84–90.

42. Olsen BS, Vaesel MT, Sojbjerg JO, et al. Lateral collateral ligament of the elbow joint: anatomy and kinematics. J Shoulder Elbow Surg 1996;5(2 Pt 1): 103–12.

43. Carrino JA, Morrison WB, Zou KH, et al. Lateral ulnar collateral ligament of the elbow: optimization

of evaluation with two-dimensional MR imaging. Radiology 2001;218(1):118–25.

44. Mehta JA, Bain GI. Posterolateral rotatory instability of the elbow. J Am Acad Orthop Surg 2004;12(6):405–15.

45. Terada N, Yamada H, Toyama Y. The appearance of the lateral ulnar collateral ligament on magnetic resonance imaging. J Shoulder Elbow Surg 2004;13(2):214–6.

46. Grafe MW, McAdams TR, Beaulieu CF, et al. Magnetic resonance imaging in diagnosis of chronic posterolateral rotatory instability of the elbow. Am J Orthop 2003;32(10):501–3 [discussion: 504].

47. Potter HG, Weiland AJ, Schatz JA, et al. Posterolateral rotatory instability of the elbow: usefulness of MR imaging in diagnosis. Radiology 1997;204(1):185–9.

48. Aoki M, Wada T, Isogai S, et al. Magnetic resonance imaging findings of refractory tennis elbows and their relationship to surgical treatment. J Shoulder Elbow Surg 2005;14(2):172–7.

49. Bennett JB. Lateral and medial epicondylitis. Hand Clin 1994;10(1):157–63.

50. Sampson S, Gerhardt M, Mandelbaum B. Platelet rich plasma injection grafts for musculoskeletal injuries: a review. Curr Rev Musculoskelet Med 2008;1(3–4):165–74.

51. Kokkalis ZT, Sotereanos DG. Biceps tendon injuries in athletes. Hand Clin 2009;25(3):347–57.

52. Festa A, Mulieri PJ, Newman JS, et al. Effectiveness of magnetic resonance imaging in detecting partial and complete distal biceps tendon rupture. J Hand Surg 2010;35(1):77–83.

53. Falchook FS, Zlatkin MB, Erbacher GE, et al. Rupture of the distal biceps tendon: evaluation with MR imaging. Radiology 1994;190(3):659–63.

54. Fitzgerald SW, Curry DR, Erickson SJ, et al. Distal biceps tendon injury: MR imaging diagnosis. Radiology 1994;191(1):203–6.

55. Karanjia ND, Stiles PJ. Cubital bursitis. J Bone Joint Surg Br 1988;70(5):832–3.

56. Skaf AY, Boutin RD, Dantas RW, et al. Bicipitoradial bursitis: MR imaging findings in eight patients and anatomic data from contrast material opacification of bursae followed by routine radiography and MR imaging in cadavers. Radiology 1999;212(1):111–6.

57. Mair SD, Isbell WM, Gill TJ, et al. Triceps tendon ruptures in professional football players. Am J Sports Med 2004;32(2):431–4.

58. Bain GI, Durrant AW. Sports-related injuries of the biceps and triceps. Clin Sports Med 2010;29(4):555–76.

59. Yeh PC, Dodds SD, Smart LR, et al. Distal triceps rupture. J Am Acad Orthop Surg 2010;18(1):31–40.

60. Kijowski R, Tuite M, Sanford M. Magnetic resonance imaging of the elbow. Part II: abnormalities of the ligaments, tendons, and nerves. Skeletal Radiol 2005;34(1):1–18.

61. Larson RL, Osternig LR. Traumatic bursitis and artificial turf. J Sports Med 1974;2(4):183–8.

62. Wasserzug O, Balicer RD, Boxman J, et al. A cluster of septic olecranon bursitis in association with infantry training. Mil Med 2011;176(1):122–4.

63. Floemer F, Morrison WB, Bongartz G, et al. MRI characteristics of olecranon bursitis. AJR Am J Roentgenol 2004;183(1):29–34.

64. Bruens ML, Dobbelaar P, Koes BW, et al. Arm injuries due to sport climbing. Ned Tijdschr Geneeskd 2008;152(33):1813–9 [in Dutch].

65. Haas JC, Meyers MC. Rock climbing injuries. Sports Med 1995;20(3):199–205.

66. Krych AJ, Kohen RB, Rodeo SA, et al. Acute brachialis muscle rupture caused by closed elbow dislocation in a professional American football player. J Shoulder Elbow Surg 2012;21(7):e1–5.

67. Griffin LY, American Orthopaedic Society for Sports Medicine. Orthopaedic knowledge update. Sports medicine. 1st edition. Rosemont (IL): American Academy of Orthopaedic Surgeons; 1994.

68. Dellon AL. Musculotendinous variations about the medial humeral epicondyle. J Hand Surg 1986;11(2):175–81.

69. Byun SD, Kim CH, Jeon IH. Ulnar neuropathy caused by an anconeus epitrochlearis: clinical and electrophysiological findings. J Hand Surg Eur Vol 2011;36(7):607–8.

70. Bladt L, Vankan Y, Demeyere A, et al. Bilateral ulnar nerve compression by anconeus epitrochlearis muscle. JBR-BTR 2009;92(2):120.

71. Andreisek G, Crook DW, Burg D, et al. Peripheral neuropathies of the median, radial, and ulnar nerves: MR imaging features. Radiographics 2006;26(5):1267–87.

72. Beltran J, Rosenberg ZS. Diagnosis of compressive and entrapment neuropathies of the upper extremity: value of MR imaging. AJR Am J Roentgenol 1994;163(3):525–31.

73. Husarik DB, Saupe N, Pfirrmann CW, et al. Elbow nerves: MR findings in 60 asymptomatic subjects. Normal anatomy, variants, and pitfalls. Radiology 2009;252(1):148–56.

74. Heithoff SJ. Cubital tunnel syndrome: ulnar nerve subluxation. J Hand Surg 2010;35(9):1556 [author reply: 1556–7].

75. Grechenig W, Mayr J, Peicha G, et al. Subluxation of the ulnar nerve in the elbow region–ultrasonographic evaluation. Acta Radiol 2003;44(6):662–4.

76. Portilla Molina AE, Bour C, Oberlin C, et al. The posterior interosseous nerve and the radial tunnel syndrome: an anatomical study. Int Orthop 1998;22(2):102–6.

77. Ferdinand BD, Rosenberg ZS, Schweitzer ME, et al. MR imaging features of radial tunnel syndrome: initial experience. Radiology 2006;240(1):161–8.

Imaging of the Pediatric Athlete: Use and Overuse

Laurie M. Lomasney, MD[a,*], Jennifer E. Lim-Dunham, MD[a], Teresa Cappello, MD[b], John Annes, MD[a]

KEYWORDS

- Chronic repetitive trauma • Stress fracture • Growth plate injury • Physeal injury • Apophysitis

KEY POINTS

- The unique patterns of sports-related trauma of the upper extremity in children and adolescents are largely caused by the fact that the open physis is the weakest part of the pediatric skeleton and thus likely to be affected in acute"use" and chronic "overuse" injuries.
- In the shoulder of the pitcher or other athlete using overhead motion, the proximal humeral physis and the tendons of the rotator cuff are particularly prone to chronic repetitive stress injury.
- In the elbow, valgus stress insults are common, especially in pitchers and gymnasts, and may manifest as apophyseal avulsion fractures, apophysitis, or osteochondritis dissicans.
- In the wrist, the distal radial physis is a common location for chronic repetitive injury.

INTRODUCTION

The noticeable increase in the number of participants in youth sports in recent decades has been paralleled by a surge in the number of associated injuries, with a reported incidence of approximately 2 million injuries annually in American high school athletes.[1] Several additional factors that contribute to the abundance of traumatic insults related to youth athletics include a progressive escalation of the level of competition, requiring increased intensity, duration, and frequency of physical activity. These elevated demands may be coupled with improper training and conditioning or inexperienced coaching, enhancing the potential for injury. Furthermore, to maximize potential for success, the young athlete commonly focuses on a single sport or specialty within a sport, necessitating repetitive motions and patterns of impact, which compound the likelihood of insult.

Many of the upper extremity injuries sustained in the skeletally immature patient are similar to those in the adult. For example, fractures of the clavicle shaft and of the forearm in football and rugby are frequently seen in adult and pediatric athletes and do not merit specific mention in this article. However, there are several distinctive traumatic insults specific to the growing athlete that form the focus of this article.

In skeletally immature athletes, the growth plate is weaker than the surrounding tendons and ligaments, and thus particularly prone to injury.[2–4] The skeleton is especially vulnerable to fracture during growth spurts because of relative bone lengthening, which results in decreased flexibility.[5] This article reviews injuries of the shoulder, elbow, and wrist that have a unique presentation in the pediatric population or that have specific relevance based on the longitudinal outcome. For each anatomic region, recommendations for imaging strategies are provided, and characteristic use and overuse injury patterns are described and illustrated. "Use" injuries typically present acutely and

[a] Department of Radiology, Stritch School of Medicine, Loyola University Medical Center, 2160 South First Avenue, Maywood, IL 60153, USA; [b] Department of Orthopaedic Surgery and Rehabilitation, Stritch School of Medicine, Loyola University Medical Center, 2160 South First Avenue, Maywood, IL 60153, USA
* Corresponding author.
E-mail address: llomasn@lumc.edu

Radiol Clin N Am 51 (2013) 215–226
http://dx.doi.org/10.1016/j.rcl.2012.09.014

are associated with an identifiable macrotraumatic event. In contrast, "overuse" injuries are associated with chronic, repetitive trauma and tend to have an insidious onset, sometimes without definable cause.[5]

SHOULDER
Use Injuries

The distribution and patterns of injuries of the shoulder region are generally predictable based on the sport activity. Acute fractures and dislocations are generally sustained in contact sports including football, rugby, and hockey. Impacts and collisions may result in adult-type insults, including fractures of the clavicle and humeral shaft, acromioclavicular (AC) separation, and glenohumeral dislocation. These injuries, which are not limited to the youth athlete, are discussed elsewhere in this issue.

One pattern of acute shoulder trauma specific to the pediatric population is the distal clavicle periosteal sleeve fracture. In the athlete at or near skeletal maturity, a direct lateral blow to the shoulder may result in AC ligamentous injury with variable frequency of ligamentous instability. In children and adolescents, however, a Salter-Harris I fracture through the physis of the distal clavicle may occur, with dissociation of the distal clavicular metaphysis from the epiphysis. In the process, the metaphysis may tear the surrounding thick periosteal sleeve and protrude cephalad, whereas the articulation between the clavicular epiphysis and acromion remains intact.[6] The standard radiographic series of the clavicle can be deceiving, sometimes showing elevation of the mineralized metaphysis with a pattern mimicking the adult pattern of AC joint separation. The natural evolution of the pediatric injury is characterized by ossification of the periosteal sleeve, gradually incorporating the distal clavicle (**Fig. 1**). Because of progressive remodeling, potential for subsequent athletic limitation or poor cosmetic outcome from this injury is low, making surgical reduction and periosteal sleeve reconstruction unnecessary in most cases.[4]

Another acute injury of the shoulder region specific to the youth athlete is a fracture of the proximal humeral physis. This is usually a Salter-Harris II fracture, and is encountered most frequently in the 11- to 15-year-old age range when the proximal humerus undergoes the most rapid growth. In contrast, children in the 5- to 11-year-old age bracket have not yet undergone their growth spurts, and subsequently, fractures of the proximal humerus in this age group most commonly affect the metaphysis without extension to the growth

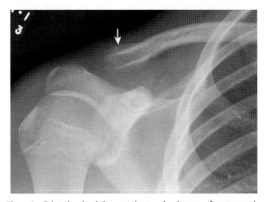

Fig. 1. Distal clavicle periosteal sleeve fracture in a 14-year-old football player. Anteroposterior (AP) radiograph of the right clavicle 4 weeks after the injury shows circumferential ossification of the periosteal sleeve (*arrow*) surrounding the distal clavicle.vc

plate.[7] Fracture of the proximal humeral physis may be superimposed on chronic metaphyseal weakening because of overuse (see later) or may be caused by a fall onto the shoulder. A standard three-view radiographic series with anteroposterior (AP), scapular Y, and axillary projections is recommended for initial imaging evaluation. Although the metaphyseal component of the fracture is easily seen, the extension of the fracture to the growth plate can be overlooked because the physeal widening may be quite subtle. The width of all portions of the physis, which is tent-shaped with the apex at the posteromedial aspect of the humerus, should be assessed for uniformity. Absence of uniformity indicates fracture extension to the growth plate. Typically, the injured physis is widened at the lateral aspect on the AP view of the shoulder (**Fig. 2**). This characteristic appearance of the Salter-Harris II fracture is thought to be partly caused by anchoring of the metaphysis to the epiphysis by the relatively thick periosteum along the posteromedial margin of the proximal humerus, driving the fracture line through the anterolateral aspect of the growth plate.[8] Secondary imaging, such as computed tomography (CT) or MR imaging, is not routinely indicated. Unless markedly displaced, fractures of the proximal humerus, with or without growth plate involvement, do not generally require open reduction because of the considerable remodeling potential of this segment of bone.[8]

Fracture through the physis at the base of the coracoid is an uncommon fracture of this age group. Because these fractures are usually the result of a direct blow, they most commonly occur in football.[9] Although the patient may complain of generalized anterior shoulder pain, pain is localized over the coracoid process. A standard three-view

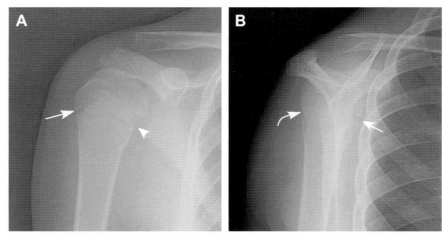

Fig. 2. Acute Salter-Harris II fracture of the proximal humerus in a 13 year old who fell on his shoulder while snowboarding. (*A*) AP radiograph of the right shoulder shows a comminuted nondisplaced fracture of the proximal humeral metaphysis, including a small medial component (*arrowhead*) that remains attached to the proximal epiphyseal fragment. The fracture extends to the growth plate, causing abnormal widening (*arrow*) of the lateral aspect of the physis. (*B*) Scapular "Y" view of the same shoulder demonstrates more clearly that the width of the physis is not uniform. Abnormal widening anteriorly (*straight arrow*) is seen compared with normal width posteriorly (*curved arrow*).

radiographic series should be obtained, with a well-positioned axillary view being the key to diagnosis. The physis at the base of the coracoid should be carefully inspected for abnormal widening, and as with many physeal injuries, a comparison view of the contralateral limb may be needed to confirm fractures with little displacement.

Overuse Injuries

Overuse injuries of the shoulder are represented by stress fractures and soft tissue injuries. Of the stress fractures, the most widely recognized example is little leaguer's shoulder. The name reflects the athletic activity most commonly associated with subacute or chronic insult to the proximal humeral physis, but any youth athlete engaged in overhead-throwing is at risk for this pathology. Excessive use, improper mechanics, and muscle imbalance all contribute to the injury.[2–4] Patients complain of diffuse shoulder pain, exacerbated by activity. A recent history of accelerated intensity of activity can often be elicited. A radiographic series, including AP projection in internal and external rotation of the humerus and an axillary view, is indicated for initial evaluation and is usually diagnostic. Classic findings include widening (possibly eccentric) of the proximal humeral physis with marginal irregularity and sclerosis, which may be detected only by comparison to the unaffected shoulder (**Fig. 3**).[3] Because the injury represents a subacute Salter-Harris I fracture, continued activity can lead to

acute fracture completion, at times associated with increased displacement.

A less familiar stress fracture in the shoulder region that may be overlooked is the vertical stress fracture of the medial or mid-shaft of the clavicle. This unique fracture is the result of young bodies literally shouldering weight beyond the capacity of their frame. During the course of training or competition, the young athlete may transport heavy bags laden with sporting equipment. If weight limits are ignored or proper carrying techniques are not observed, the child repeatedly slings the load over the same shoulder day after day, resulting in clavicular bone fatigue.[10] The athlete then experiences increasing pain and limited athletic achievement. The plain radiograph is a simple diagnostic tool to visualize vertical sclerosis of the medial or mid-shaft of the clavicle indicative of the subacute fracture. The abnormality may be subtle, because the fracture is rarely displaced, and the images must therefore be scrutinized carefully to avoid missing this important diagnosis (**Fig. 4**).

The soft tissue structures about the shoulder are especially prone to overuse injuries. The repetitive overhead motion of the upper extremity executed in such sports as swimming, tennis, and throwing are common sources of trauma to the tendons and muscles, most frequently the rotator cuff. Internal impingement secondary to confinement by the humeral head and posterior glenoid, and powerful tensile forces of the muscles themselves, result in excessive stress and tendonitis in the

A   **B**

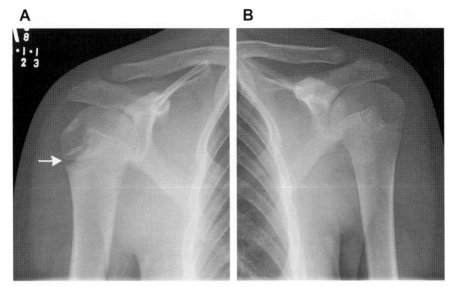

Fig. 3. Chronic right proximal humeral physeal stress fracture (little leaguer's shoulder) in a 14-year-old right-hand dominant pitcher. (*A*) AP radiograph of the affected right shoulder shows abnormal widening and marginal irregularity of the lateral aspect of the growth plate (*arrow*). (*B*) AP comparison radiograph of the unaffected left shoulder shows normal width and well-defined margins of the intact physis.

rotator cuff, specifically the posterior fibers of the supraspinatus tendon and anterior fibers of the infraspinatus tendon.[11] The patient complains of anterolateral pain exacerbated with continued training. Radiographs are occasionally helpful to identify anomalous bony anatomy contributing to impingement, including a hooked anterior acromion or os acromiale. MR imaging is the most commonly used imaging test for diagnosis of rotator cuff tendinosis. Although multiplanar imaging should be completed, coronal proton density (PD) and T2-weighted images are most beneficial to visualize the supraspinatus and infraspinatus tendons. Tendon thickening with intermediate signal on PD imaging, but without high T2 signal, confirms the diagnosis of tendinopathy (**Fig. 5**). Less commonly, injury may be more severe with high T2 signal, which indicates partial- or full-thickness tear of the tendon. MR arthrography is not necessary unless there is also a clinical concern of glenohumeral instability.

An alternative modality to MR imaging is ultrasound (US). With a trained operator, US interrogation of the rotator cuff can provide accurate results for determination of tendinosis. With US, the individual tendons of the rotator cuff can be inspected for possible distortion of internal architecture or thickening associated with tendinopathy. Additionally, focal bursal or capsular defects, partial thickness tears, or less commonly full-thickness defects with or without tendon retraction can be seen. An advantage of the real-time capability of US is that dynamic maneuvers can be performed to evaluate for supraspinatus impingement by the bony confine of the supraspinatus outlet or acromial enthesophytes. A study of 71 patients by Teefey and colleagues[12] showed identical accuracy of 87% for MR imaging and US in discriminating partial- and full-thickness tears, with arthroscopy used as the gold standard. However, high-quality US is not consistently offered at clinical offices and imaging centers. Furthermore, if alternative diagnoses, such as a labral tear, are under consideration, MR imaging can provide a more global evaluation than can US.

ELBOW
Use Injuries

Elbow dislocation is usually sustained as an impact injury and presents immediately for clinical

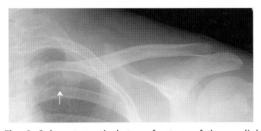

Fig. 4. Subacute vertical stress fracture of the medial clavicle. AP radiograph of the left clavicle shows linear lucency surrounded by faint sclerosis (*arrow*).

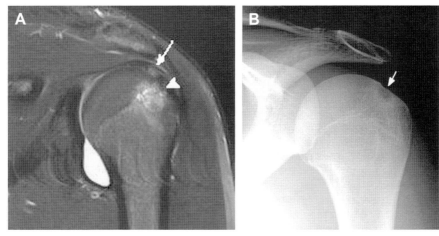

Fig. 5. Shoulder internal impingement causing rotator cuff tendinopathy in a left-hand dominant 18-year-old pitcher. (*A*) T2 fat-saturated coronal MR arthrogram image of left shoulder shows intermediate signal in the posterior supraspinatus tendon (*arrow*) with reactive cystic changes and surrounding high signal bone marrow edema in the posterolateral humerus (*arrowhead*) at the site of supraspinatus tendon attachment. (*B*) AP radiograph of the same shoulder shows subcortical cyst (*arrow*) corresponding to MR imaging finding.

evaluation. Gymnasts and football players are at particular risk, given the high frequency of fall and impact trauma.[5] Most dislocations are posterior or posterolateral in direction, and may be associated with medial epicondyle avulsion fracture in the patient with open physes. In the older athlete with closed physes, there may be small avulsion fragments at the medial collateral ligament attachment to the medial epicondyle. A standard radiographic series should be adequate to diagnose the acute dislocation, generally showing complete dislocation of radius and ulna.

Radiographs are essential for evaluation after closed reduction of the dislocation. In the skeletally immature athlete, postreduction radiographs are critical not only for confirmation of complete reduction, but also for detection of complications from an associated medial epicondyle fracture. With coincident valgus stress at the time of dislocation, the medial epicondyle apophysis in the patient with open physes may be avulsed and displaced distally. On closed reduction, the apophysis can become entrapped between the trochlea and ulna (**Fig. 6**). Well-positioned frontal, oblique, and

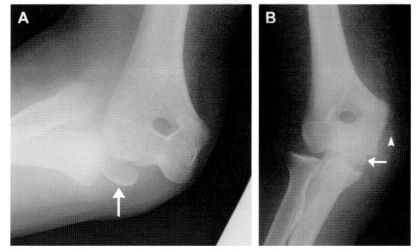

Fig. 6. Elbow dislocation with associated medial epicondyle fracture in a 15-year-old wrestler. (*A*) Oblique radiograph of the right elbow shows the dislocation and the avulsed, displaced medial epicondyle apophysis (*arrow*). (*B*) Oblique radiograph after closed reduction of the dislocation shows that the medial epicondyle fracture fragment (*arrow*) remains entrapped between the trochlea and the ulna. Tiny fracture fragments (*arrowhead*) arising from the medial epicondyle metaphysis are also seen.

lateral radiographs should be inspected carefully. Secondary imaging with CT or MR imaging is not usually indicated.

Isolated acute medial epicondyle avulsion fractures, without associated elbow dislocation, are the result of sudden tension from contraction of the flexor-pronator muscle mass. In the younger athlete, the entire epicondylar apophysis may be avulsed.[13] Radiographs are the indicated primary imaging modality. A three-view series with AP, internal oblique, and lateral views is recommended, with the abnormality best profiled on the internal oblique view. Widening of the physis with sharp margination of the opposed bone margins and localized soft tissue swelling are often seen. More severe injuries show progressive displacement of the epicondyle, usually retracted caudal toward the joint line (**Fig. 7**). Many of these injuries can be treated conservatively with immobilization, although open reduction and internal fixation may be indicated if the fragment is significantly displaced or if the child participates in upper extremity weight-bearing activity, such as gymnastics or wrestling.[1]

In the older athlete with closed physes, the acute fracture of the medial epicondyle may manifest as small bony avulsion fragments at the attachment of the ulnar collateral ligament attachment or the flexor-pronator bundle rather than as a fragment encompassing the entire apophysis (**Fig. 8**).[13] If clinically appropriate, valgus stress views of the affected side and the contralateral side (for comparison) can be obtained. Asymmetric medial joint line opening greater than 2 mm suggests instability, which can predispose

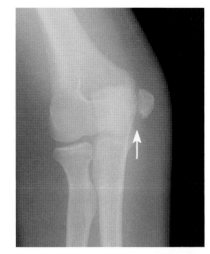

Fig. 8. Acute medial epicondyle avulsion fracture in a 14-year-old football player. AP radiograph of the right elbow shows abnormally widened medial epicondyle growth plate (*arrow*), with abrupt bony interface.

the young patient to premature osteoarthritis and chronic disability.[14] For those patients unresponsive to initial conservative management of rest and immobilization, MR imaging can be valuable to further characterize the pattern of injury. PD and T2-weighted fat-suppressed coronal plane imaging with anatomic arm position, elbow flexed 15 degrees, and scan plane parallel to the humerus is effective for maximizing visualization of the anterior band of the ulnar collateral ligament.

Supracondylar fractures in the young athlete are no different in mechanism, imaging algorithm, treatment, or potential sequelae compared with the nonathlete.[5] As reiterated throughout the imaging literature, a precisely positioned lateral view is critical for identification of an elevated posterior elbow fat pad, which has a significant association with the presence of a subtle or occult intra-articular fracture.[14] Verification of articulation between radial head and capitellum in all projections and confirmation of intact anterior humeral line should be completed.

Overuse Injuries

Valgus stress overuse injuries of the elbow, which frequently take the form of medial epicondylar apophysitis, are especially common in the adolescent pitcher, giving rise to the term "little leaguer's elbow." The late cocking and early acceleration phases of the throwing action result in distraction on the medial side of the elbow with simultaneous compression on the lateral side.[13] Distraction stresses in the medial compartment may manifest

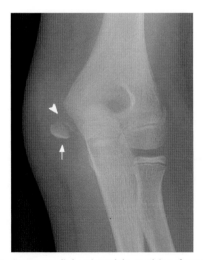

Fig. 7. Acute medial epicondyle avulsion fracture in a 10-year-old gymnast. Oblique radiograph of the left elbow shows that the medial epicondylar apophysis (*arrow*), along with a thin rim of metaphysis (*arrowhead*), is avulsed and displaced distally.

as medial epicondylar apophysitis or ulnar collateral ligament insufficiency. With continued valgus stress, compressive injury in the lateral compartment can also occur, resulting in avascular necrosis of the capitellum in the younger pitcher and osteochondritis dissecans (OCD) of the radial head or capitellum in the older adolescent.[1] Various pitches have differing patterns of stress and potential points of injury, with breaking pitches, especially sliders, having an 86% increase in risk for elbow pain.[1] This association is so compelling that the American Sports Medicine Institute USA Baseball Medical and Advisory Committee developed recommendations in 1996 for cumulative pitch counts and days of interval rest between pitches to reduce elbow and shoulder injuries.[15]

Plain radiography is the primary imaging modality used to evaluate the athlete with medial joint line pain. Medial epicondylar apophysitis can be considered a subacute or chronic Salter-Harris I stress fracture through the physis of the medial epicondyle, and radiographs accordingly show physeal widening and irregularity with sclerosis of the opposing bone margins (**Fig. 9**). Relative overgrowth of the apophyseal fragment secondary to regional hyperemia may be seen. In the earliest stages, comparison with the asymptomatic extremity may be needed to confirm the pathology. If radiographs are indeterminate, an appropriate course of action may include cessation of activity followed by reimaging in 2 to 3 months to evaluate for evolution, such as improved demarcation of fracture margins or fusion of the injured physis.

In cases where cautious observation and training limitation is not desirable, MR imaging may be used as a problem-solving tool. Axial and coronal images with T2-weighted imaging are beneficial to see soft tissue and bony changes. High T2-signal, especially fluid intensity, along the physis with marginal bone marrow edema pattern is characteristic. In some cases, the edema may be focused entirely within the medial epicondyle, such as when the flexor-pronator muscle mass is responsible for chronic tension injury. Joint effusion is not expected, because the medial epicondyle is extra-articular. One benefit of MR imaging is interrogation of regional structures such as the ulnar collateral ligament, which may demonstrate associated tear or laxity (**Fig. 10**).

Isolated injuries to the ulnar collateral ligament are relatively uncommon in the athlete with open physis because the physis represents the weaker point. However, most of these injuries when seen are related to overuse. The standard radiographic

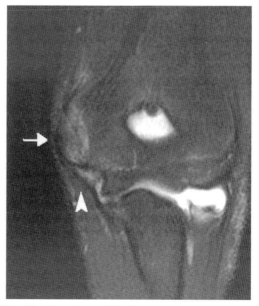

Fig. 10. Chronic medial elbow injury secondary to valgus stress in a 12-year-old right-hand dominant pitcher. Coronal T2 fat-saturated MR arthrogram image of the right elbow shows high signal bone marrow edema in the medial epicondyle apophysis, adjacent growth plate, and metaphysis (*arrow*). Intermediate-high signal at the humeral attachment of the anterior band of the ulnar collateral ligament (*arrowhead*) indicates a partial tear.

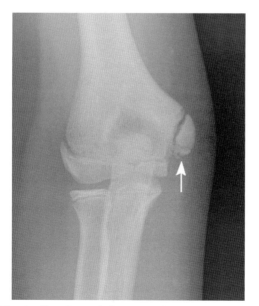

Fig. 9. Chronic medial epicondyle apophysitis and physeal injury secondary to valgus stress (little leaguer's elbow) in a 13-year-old right-hand dominant baseball player. AP radiograph of the right elbow shows abnormal fragmentation of the medial epicondyle (*arrow*) with excessive widening, irregularity, and sclerosis of the adjacent growth plate.

series is usually not informative. Stress radiographs may be of benefit but must include views of the contralateral extremity to account for variable but normal pediatric ligamentous laxity.[13] MR imaging may provide valuable information in cases recalcitrant to conservative management or with gross clinical instability. Traditional MR imaging emphasizing coronal plane imaging (high-resolution PD images or T2-weighted fat-suppressed images) is usually sufficient to visualize the dominant stabilizer, the anterior band of the ulnar collateral ligament. Abnormal intermediate PD or high T2 signal traversing the ligament, especially at the humeral attachment, is indicative of a tear. MR arthrography may provide additional information in the older adolescent, because intra-articular contrast distention improves sensitivity for detection of partial-thickness injuries.[16]

Static and dynamic US may also be used to evaluate the integrity of the anterior band of the ulnar collateral ligament. Imaging is completed in 30 degrees of elbow flexion to provide optimal profiling of the anterior band (paralleling the flexed position for MR imaging). Static imaging shows anatomic detail of the anterior band including continuity from the medial humeral epicondyle to the sublime tubercle; morphology (thickness and definition); and character (presence of internal calcifications). Dynamic imaging includes measure of the medial joint line width at rest and with application of valgus stress.[17] Comparative imaging of the contralateral, asymptomatic limb is completed to provide an internal standard, especially for the dynamic imaging, thus taking into account the ligamentous laxity of youth. In a study by Nazarian and colleagues,[17] valgus stress US showed an average medial joint line widening of 1.2 mm more on the dominant arm compared with the nonpitching arm of major baseball league pitchers.

Compressive lateral compartment injuries may be coincident with medial injury in children with elbow valgus stress insult. These injuries include Panner disease, which represents devascularization of the capitellum, and which is usually seen in young children in the 4- to 9-year-old age group.[1] Clinical complaints are usually vague, with gradual onset of lateral pain and loss of extension in the dominant throwing arm in pitchers (the most commonly associated activity), or in either arm in the gymnast.[5] On plain radiographs, the secondary ossification center of the capitellum may be small and sclerotic in the prepubescent youth with global devascularization. In the older adolescent athlete, focal subacute osteochondral lesions of the capitellum and radial head are more frequent than global epiphyseal fragmentation (Fig. 11).[1,13] Pain and stiffness are the most

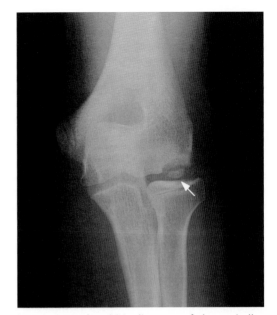

Fig. 11. Osteochondritis dissecans of the capitellum secondary to elbow valgus stress in a 14-year-old left-hand dominant pitcher. AP radiograph of the left elbow shows fragmented osteochondral lesion at the capitellum (arrow). The fragments appear separated from the donor site, although articular cartilage integrity cannot be determined on radiographs. Note also mild radial head overgrowth.

frequent symptoms, with frank locking when the isolated fragment has progressed to a loose body in the joint.

Radiographs are important for characterization of the capitellum and radial head. Occasionally, radiographs may show overgrowth of the radial head as a stress response.[18] Sclerosis, fragmentation, and collapse of the capitellum or radial head may be seen in some cases of devascularization. However, multicentric ossifications centers in the capitellum may confuse the diagnosis for Panner disease. Small OCD lesions may be obscured or overlooked on radiographs. CT can be used to confirm equivocal radiographic findings, although articular cartilage integrity and articular collapse are not well characterized without the benefit of intra-articular injection of iodinated contrast. In addition, CT delivers a very small but perhaps unnecessary radiation dose. Therefore, MR imaging or MR arthrography is recommended to further evaluate integrity of the secondary ossification center or the osteochondral lesion. MR imaging in the presence of native joint effusion or iatrogenic capsular distention is extremely sensitive and specific not only for identification of OCD lesions, but also for evaluation of fragment stability, which is a major factor impacting choice of arthroscopic versus conservative management.[19–22] The cartilaginous surface is normally smooth, and an articular cartilage cleft profiled by joint fluid is abnormal. Additionally, if fluid completely encompasses a bone fragment, the fragment is at increased risk for mobilization, and arthroscopic stabilization or debridement would be considered.

Lateral joint line stress at the elbow is greatest for athletes engaged in racket sports, although the follow-through phase for overhead throwing athletes also produces substantial lateral stress.[13] In racket sports, repeated wrist extension is completed by the strong pull of the extensors originating at the lateral epicondyle. Therefore, overuse and repetitive training may result in a physeal injury pattern similar to that described for the medial apophysis, although in a younger age group, given the earlier fusion of the lateral epicondyle physis compared with the medial epicondyle physis. The patient complains of lateral joint line pain and decreased power. Because the diagnosis is usually made based on clinical findings, radiographs are rarely indicated, but may show physeal widening and irregularity.[13]

Posterior compartment injuries are uncommon in children, but when they occur, usually take the form of overuse trauma to the olecranon. These insults occur in the throwing athlete during the deceleration and the follow-through phases from repetitive elbow extension and tension traction overload forces secondary to contraction of the triceps, which inserts on the olecranon.[4,13] Similar injuries may also be seen in gymnasts,[23] wrestlers, and hockey players. In the younger athlete with unfused physes, olecranon apophysitis and olecranon OCD, which are best demonstrated with MR imaging, are considerations (**Fig. 12**). Radiographs are most useful in the older athlete at or near the time of growth plate fusion. In these patients, avulsion fractures of the olecranon apophysis may be seen, manifesting as physeal widening, marginal fraying, and possibly apophysis sclerosis or fragmentation. A superimposed acute completed fracture may occur with continued throwing activity,[14] especially with increased ossification of the apophysis.[23] The presence of multiple ossification centers is a common normal variant in the olecranon, and therefore, comparison with radiographs of the contralateral elbow is often helpful.

After the olecranon physis is fused, injury in the overhead throwing athlete may be soft tissue based, paralleling the adult pattern, with posterolateral synovial hypertrophy and impingement. Symptoms include pain and limited range of motion. Eccentric articular cartilage wear also results in marginal osteophytosis, provoking further synovial injury and impingement. The standard radiographic series

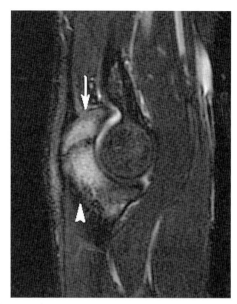

Fig. 12. Olecranon apophysitis in a 16-year-old martial arts student. Sagittal T2 fat-saturated MR image of the elbow shows abnormally increased olecranon apophysis bone marrow signal (*arrow*), which also extends into the adjacent proximal ulnar metaphysis (*arrowhead*). (*Courtesy of* Kate Feinstein, MD, University of Chicago, Chicago, IL.)

is generally not helpful, although a cubital tunnel view profiling the posterior joint line and olecranon may reveal osteophytosis and loose bodies.

WRIST
Use Injuries

The wrist is vulnerable to acute injury in many athletic activities, but is particularly susceptible to trauma in sports where the athlete regularly falls, such as football and snowboarding. The distal radius is a common site of fracture, with the precise anatomic localization dependent on the age of the child. In the younger child, the metaphysis of the distal radius is most prone to injury, whereas in the older adolescent, the physis of the distal radius is most likely to fracture, commonly in a Salter-Harris I or II pattern.[4]

The scaphoid is the most commonly fractured carpal bone in children. In past decades, up to 87% of scaphoid fractures in children involved the distal pole (**Fig. 13**).[4,24] Complications from distal pole fractures are rare, and thus these fractures rarely require operative treatment. More recently, the injury pattern in children has shifted such that most scaphoid fractures now involve the waist, identical to the adult pattern. This change is thought to be secondary to the higher energy impacts, previously reserved for adults, sustained by today's young athlete.[4,25]

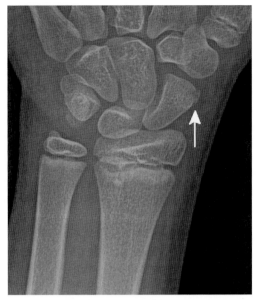

Fig. 13. Oblique radiograph of the left wrist shows acute fracture of the distal pole of the scaphoid (*arrow*) in a 10-year-old volleyball player.

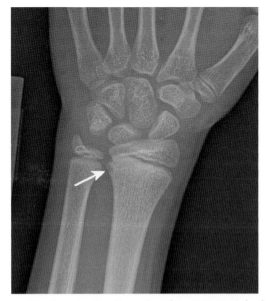

Fig. 14. Chronic repetitive injury (gymnast's wrist) of the distal radial physis in an 11-year-old gymnast. Oblique radiograph of the left wrist shows eccentric widening and marginal sclerosis of the growth plate of the distal radius, with development of a reactive cyst in the metaphysis (*arrow*).

Overuse Injuries

Of the overuse injuries of the pediatric athlete, the gymnast's wrist is the best described, representing a spectrum from evolving bony injury to permanent growth disturbances and ligamentous injuries. Original descriptions focused on chronic repetitive axial loading injury to the distal radial physis secondary to the practice of supporting the entire body weight on the upper extremities in gymnastics. Radiographs are useful for documenting widening and loss of definition of the affected distal radial physis; they may also demonstrate sclerosis and irregularity at the margins of the physis, and secondary reactive cyst formation at the metaphyseal margin of the affected growth plate (**Fig. 14**).[23,24] Over time, foci of interposed cartilaginous ingrowth and bridging may develop,[26–28] with the potential for either partial or complete bony bar at the physis. Premature physeal fusion of the radius may result in relative ulnar lengthening because of continued, normal ulnar growth.[26,28–31] Studies have confirmed relatively exaggerated ulnar lengthening in gymnasts in the 12- to 18-year-old age range, with negative ulnar variance measuring only −1.8 mm compared with the more pronounced normal negative ulnar variance of −2.2 to −2.3 mm in the general population for this age group (**Fig. 15**).[26]

Ulnar-positive variance and continued repetitive axial load places the athlete at an increased risk of additional secondary pathologies including

lunate chondromalacia and triangular fibrocartilage complex tear.[4] Radiographs are not typically useful for making these secondary diagnoses. MR imaging is the indicated imaging modality to evaluate focal

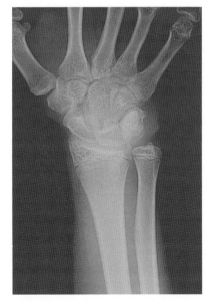

Fig. 15. Sequela of chronic repetitive injury of the distal radial physis in a 13-year-old gymnast. Posteroanterior radiograph of the right wrist shows exaggerated lengthening of the ulna relative to the radius, which is the result of deficient longitudinal growth of the radius.

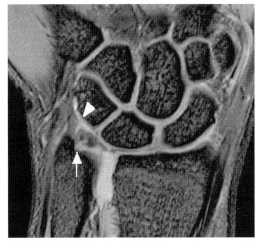

Fig. 16. Tears of the triangular fibrocartilage complex in a 20-year-old former gymnast. Coronal gradient echo fat-saturated MR image shows high signal triangular fibrocartilage complex tears at its proximal surface (*arrow*) and near its attachment to the ulnar styloid (*arrowhead*). Also noted is distal radioulnar joint effusion.

cartilaginous defects at the lunate and diagnose the spectrum of triangular fibrocartilage complex injuries (**Fig. 16**).

SUMMARY

Recent years have witnessed a steady rise in the number of sports-related upper extremity injuries involving the shoulder, elbow, and wrists in children and adolescents. Correspondingly, radiologists are increasingly likely to encounter these abnormalities during the course of their daily practice. These injuries, which can be seen in the setting of acute "use" trauma or chronic "overuse" trauma, tend to occur in predictable and recognizable patterns, primarily related to the presence of open growth plates and apophyseal ossification centers in the pediatric population. Many of these injuries have a characteristic imaging appearance, often best evaluated with plain radiographs. If interpretation of the plain film is in doubt, radiography of the contralateral side can be invaluable as a problem-solving tool, but should be used judiciously. If necessary, secondary imaging with MR imaging, with or without arthrography, and CT may be beneficial in selected clinical scenarios.

REFERENCES

1. Mariscalco MW, Saluan P. Upper extremity injuries in the adolescent athlete. Sports Med Arthrosc 2011; 19(1):17–26.

2. Frank J, Kramer D, Kocher M. Shoulder injuries in the pediatric athlete. In: Song KM, editor. OKU, Orthopaedic Knowledge Update. Pediatrics 4. Rosemont (IL): American Academy of Orthopaedic Surgeons; 2011. p. 429–36.

3. Carson WG Jr, Gasser SI. Little leaguer's shoulder. A report of 23 cases. Am J Sports Med 1998;26(4): 575–80.

4. Kocher MS, Waters PM, Micheli LJ. Upper extremity injuries in the paediatric athlete. Sports Med 2000; 30(2):117–35.

5. Shanmugam C, Maffulli N. Sports injuries in children. Br Med Bull 2008;86:33–57.

6. Ogden JA. Distal clavicular physeal injury. Clin Orthop Relat Res 1984;(188):68–73.

7. Kwon Y, Sarwark J. Proximal humerus, scapula and clavicle. In: Rockwood CA, Wilkins KE, Beaty JH, et al, editors. Rockwood and Wilkins' fractures in children. 5th edition. Philadelphia: Lippincott Williams & Wilkins; 2001. p. 744.

8. Mooney JF, Webb LX. Fractures and dislocations about the shoulder. In: Green NE, Swiontkowski MF, editors. Skeletal trauma in children. 4th edition. Philadelphia: Saunders/Elsevier; 2008. Available at: http://www.Mdconsult.com/books/page.do?eid=4-u1.0-B978-1-4160-4900-5.10010-X–s0440&isbn=978-1-4160-4900-5&uniqId=332799267-2#4-u1.0-B978-1-4160-4900-5.10010-X–s0440; 2008. Online resource (xviii, 709 p). Accessed April 29, 2012.

9. Davis KW. Imaging pediatric sports injuries: upper extremity. Radiol Clin North Am 2010;48(6):1199–211.

10. Krakowski FM. Young athletes get injuries too. Available at: http://www.scpgajrtour.com/2011/10/young.athletes.get.injuries.too/. Accessed April 27, 2012.

11. Giaroli EL, Major NM, Higgins LD. MRI of internal impingement of the shoulder. AJR Am J Roentgenol 2005;185(4):925–9.

12. Teefey SA, Rubin DA, Middleton WD, et al. Detection and quantification of rotator cuff tears. J Bone Joint Surg Am 2004;86:708–16.

13. Chen FS, Diaz VA, Loebenberg M, et al. Shoulder and elbow injuries in the skeletally immature athlete. J Am Acad Orthop Surg 2005;13(3):172–85.

14. Cox D, Sonin A. The elbow and forearm. In: Rogers LF, editor. Radiology of skeletal trauma. 3rd edition. Philadelphia: Churchill Livingstone; 2002. p. 683.

15. Andrews J, Fleisig G. Little league regulation: protecting young pitchers' arms. Available at: http://www.littleleague.org/Assets/old_assets/media/pitch_count_publication_2008.pdf. Accessed April 29, 2012.

16. Steinbach LS, Palmer WE, Schweitzer ME. Special focus session. MR arthrography. Radiographics 2002;22(5):1223–46.

17. Nazarian LN, McShane JM, Ciccotti MG, et al. Dynamic ultrasound of the anterior band of the ulnar collateral ligament of the elbow in asymptomatic major league baseball pitchers. Radiology 2003;227:149–54.

18. Micheli LJ, Fehlandt AF Jr. Overuse injuries to tendons and apophyses in children and adolescents. Clin Sports Med 1992;11(4):713–26.

19. Mirzayan R. Clinical evaluation of the patient with a chondral injury. In: Mirzayan R, editor. Cartilage injury in the athlete. New York: Thieme; 2006. p. 47–9.

20. Baker CL III, Romeo AA, Baker CL Jr. Osteochondritis dissecans of the capitellum. Am J Sports Med 2010;38(9):1917–28.

21. Kramer J, Stiglbauer R, Engel A, et al. MR contrast arthrography (MRA) in osteochondrosis dissecans. J Comput Assist Tomogr 1992;16(2):254–60.

22. Maffulli N, Chan D, Aldridge MJ. Overuse injuries of the olecranon in young gymnasts. J Bone Joint Surg Br 1992;74(2):305–8.

23. DiFiori JP, Caine DJ, Malina RM. Wrist pain, distal radial physeal injury, and ulnar variance in the young gymnast. Am J Sports Med 2006;34(5):840–9.

24. Carter SR, Aldridge MJ. Stress injury of the distal radial growth plate. J Bone Joint Surg Br 1988;70(5): 834–6.

25. Gholson JJ, Bae DS, Zurakowski D, et al. Scaphoid fractures in children and adolescents: contemporary injury patterns and factors influencing time to union. J Bone Joint Surg Am 2011;93(13):1210–9.

26. Dwek JR, Cardoso F, Chung CB. MR imaging of overuse injuries in the skeletally immature gymnast: spectrum of soft-tissue and osseous lesions in the hand and wrist. Pediatr Radiol 2009;39(12): 1310–6.

27. Ecklund K, Jaramillo D. Patterns of premature physeal arrest: MR imaging of 111 children. Am J Roentgenol 2002;178(4):967–72.

28. Jaramillo D, Laor T, Zaleske DJ. Indirect trauma to the growth plate: results of MR imaging after epiphyseal and metaphyseal injury in rabbits. Radiology 1993;187(1):171–8.

29. Chang CY, Shih C, Penn IW, et al. Wrist injuries in adolescent gymnasts of a Chinese opera school: radiographic survey. Radiology 1995; 195(3):861–4.

30. De Smet L, Claessens A, Lefevre J, et al. Gymnast wrist: an epidemiologic survey of ulnar variance and stress changes of the radial physis in elite female gymnasts. Am J Sports Med 1994;22(6): 846–50.

31. Mandelbaum BR, Bartolozzi AR, Davis CA, et al. Wrist pain syndrome in the gymnast. Pathogenetic, diagnostic, and therapeutic considerations. Am J Sports Med 1989;17(3):305–17.

Magnetic Resonance Arthrography of the Upper Extremity

Laurie M. Lomasney, MD[a,*], Haemi Choi, MD[b], Neeru Jayanthi, MD[c,d]

KEYWORDS

- MR arthrography • Techniques • Upper extremity

KEY POINTS

Shoulder Arthrography

- Key indications: partial thickness capsular surface tears, labrum, postrotator cuff repair.
- Three approaches can be used including 2 anterior (rotator cuff interval and subscapularis) and 1 posterior approach.
- The addition of lidocaine for articular fluids allows for a diagnostic challenge.

Elbow Arthrography

- Key indications: ulnar collateral ligament tears, osteochondral defect, loose body.
- Three approaches may be used including direct lateral, posterior paralateral, and transtriceps tendon.

Wrist Arthrography

- Key indications: intrinsic ligament injury, chondral injuries, triangular fibrocartilage complex tear.
- Unicompartmental injection into the radiocarpal joint is more common than tricompartmental injection for magnetic resonance arthrography.

The introduction of magnetic resonance (MR) imaging to the imaging armamentarium has allowed detailed interrogation of the musculoskeletal elements contributing to stability and function of the joints of the upper extremities. Direct visualization of previously unobservable and/or unfamiliar structures has driven both discovery and innovation. With this tool, imagers and clinicians have gained significant insight into diagnosis and treatment options for athletes.

Using basic imaging sequences, MR imaging excels as a tool for assessment of internal derangement and injury to the musculoskeletal complex of the joints of the upper extremities. Although potentially pathologic, the presence of a joint effusion is a bonus, providing distention to lift and separate juxtaposed structures as well as providing an improved profile of structures such as ligaments and tendons. In contrast to the knee, however, upper extremity joints normally have little capsular fluid even when injured. Subtle injuries with clinical significance can be missed. There is some evidence that indirect MR arthrography (intravenous injection of gadolinium with

[a] Department of Radiology, Loyola University Medical Center, 2160 South First Avenue, Maywood, IL 60153, USA; [b] Department of Family Medicine, Loyola University Medical Center, Room 260, Building 54, 2160 South First Avenue, Maywood, IL 60153, USA; [c] Department of Family Medicine, Loyola University Medical Center, 2160 South First Avenue, Maywood, IL 60153, USA; [d] Department of Orthopedic Surgery and Rehabilitation, Loyola University Medical Center, 2160 South First Avenue, Maywood, IL 60153, USA
* Corresponding author.
E-mail address: llomasn@lumc.edu

Radiol Clin N Am 51 (2013) 227–237
http://dx.doi.org/10.1016/j.rcl.2012.11.001

radiologic.theclinics.com

MR imaging after a 20-minute delay) is a valuable technique for evaluation of internal derangement including labral injury.[1] However, imaging after direct intra-articular injection provides excellent sensitivity and specificity for imaging several patterns of injury, providing both capsular distention and a structure profile.[2] Routine injection for all examinations is not advocated. Prospective consideration for joint distention, however, should be given for specific indications as discussed in this article.

A variety of techniques can be used for successful injection of joints. Similarly, the literature is replete with options for MR imaging sequences after intra-articular injection, because the parameters must be modified to accommodate the injection agent. This article addresses specific techniques to administer the articular fluid and basic imaging considerations are presented.

SHOULDER

Shoulder pain and instability may be the result of a pathologic condition in numerous structures of the shoulder, most notably the rotator cuff and the glenoid labrum. Clinical history and physical examination are essential to determine the cause and decide on operative versus nonoperative management. Imaging is used to clarify or confirm the cause of shoulder dysfunction. Routine MR imaging without intra-articular injection may be satisfactory for evaluation of the shoulder in certain scenarios including evaluation of rotator cuff injuries in an elderly patient with high-riding humeral head on radiographs. However, a young athlete presenting with deep aching shoulder pain (particularly with overhead activity) that has clicking and a sense of instability may have a labral tear. There are several maneuvers performed on physical examination to help with diagnosis such as the O'Brien test, the Speed test, and the anterior slide test, but specificity and sensitivity are low in diagnosis, indicating the need for an MR arthrogram for confirmation.[3,4] Articular distention is advocated to provide an optimum profile of the fibrous glenoid labrum and the articular surface of the rotator cuff tendons.

MR arthrography has been shown to be superior to routine MR for detection of partial thickness undersurface tears of the rotator cuff and glenoid labrum tears, especially superior labral anterior to posterior (SLAP) labral injuries. The literature reports that up to 10% of partial and full thickness rotator cuff tears do not show a characteristic high T2-weighted signal at the defects on routine MR imaging, possibly because of low signal granulation tissue filling the defect.[5] After articular

distention, however, high T1-weighted signal with gadolinium opacifies the tear.[6] Articular distention is also beneficial for evaluation of rotator cuff integrity after surgical repair. Between susceptibility artifacts and scar/granulation tissue, intrasubstance and marginal signal abnormalities may make interpretation of signal abnormalities challenging. Bursal distention with gadolinium after intra-articular injection or gadolinium intravasation within the substance of rotator cuff tendons aids interpretation.[7]

Technique

A variety of techniques have been described for introduction of fluids into the glenohumeral capsule. Ultimately, the optimum technique is the one with which the proceduralist is most familiar and has completed most frequently. However, the rotator cuff interval approach is commonly used and has several advantages. A shorter injection needle is used with a simplistic direct anterior-posterior approach, taking advantage of the capacious capsular overlap of the humeral head. Few structures are in the trajectory of the needle path.[8]

Rotator cuff interval approach
Preparatory materials
> Gadolinium diluted 1:250: 9 mL
> Lidocaine 1%: 4 mL
> Iodinated contrast, 300 mg/L: <5 mL; with short connector tube
> Lidocaine 1%: local anesthesia
> 38-mm (1.5-inch) 22G spinal needle

The patient is positioned supine on a table with the humerus neutral or mildly internally rotated (**Fig. 1**). The desired injection site is localized at the superomedial humeral head, approximately at the level of the superior glenoid, 3 mm from

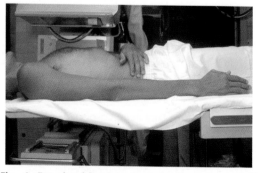

Fig. 1. For shoulder injection via the rotator cuff interval, the patient is positioned supine, arm extended to the side. The humerus is positioned in neutral or mild internal rotation.

the medial humeral cortex. After sterile preparation and local anesthesia, the spinal needle is advanced perpendicular to horizontal until bone impact. The short length of the needle is especially advantageous when completing this examination with a trainee because this allows the supervisor to visually perceive the depth of needle placement; the needle would rarely be hubbed if in the proper position. The intra-articular position is confirmed with infusion of less than 1 mL of iodinated contrast under fluoroscopic observation, with contrast generally flowing briskly into the subcoracoid bursa (**Fig. 2**). Contrast preferentially flowing into the subacromial/subdeltoid bursa may indicate incorrect needle position or a full thickness rotator cuff tear (**Fig. 3**). If the needle is in the proper position, 9 mL of dilute gadolinium (1:250) mixed with 4 mL of lidocaine 1% are injected. The needle is removed and appropriate hemostasis applied.

Caudal subscapularis approach

For this approach, the patient is positioned supine. In contrast to the superomedial approach, the humerus is positioned in neutral or mild external rotation. A point is localized over the inferior humeral head/glenohumeral space. The needle is positioned 1.5 cm lateral to the destination mark and angled medially to the projected space.[10,11] Some degree of three-dimensional perception is required to accommodate varying patient size. Generally, a 76-mm (3-inch) 22G spinal needle is needed because of the obliquity. If the needle tip is intracapsular, iodinated contrast usually flows briskly into the axillary pouch (**Fig. 4**). The gadolinium/lidocaine ratio and the quantity of contrast infused are identical to the superomedial approach.

Posterior The posterior approach is routinely used in a clinical setting where fluoroscopy is unavailable. Although less commonly used by imagers,

---

Tips and Tricks:

1. Place a towel behind the shoulder to stabilize but not reposition the humeral head; this may decrease discomfort especially for patients with posterior injury or instability.

2. In the event of contrast opacifying the subacromial bursa, consider internally and externally rotating the humerus under fluoroscopic observation to visualize the flow of contrast material. If the contrast migrates medially to the cover articular cartilage of the humeral head, the intra-articular position is confirmed and the injection can be completed.

3. If the iodinated test contrast preferentially opacifies the bicipetal tendon sheath, gadolinium injection can be completed successfully, but the infusion should be slow and gentle to allow contrast to flow cephalad to the articular capsule and avoid nonadverse but suboptimal rupture of the sheath. Consider telling the patient they may feel pressure over the anterior upper arm.

4. Do not overdistend the capsule because this may result in physiologic extravasation at the subscapularis bursa. Although not detrimental to the patient because this is the physiologic route of decompression, the benefits of capsular distention are negated. Generally, 13 mL of solution provide an appropriate balance of distention and capsular integrity, although fluid must never be forcefully injected under resistance because developmental variations and surgical modifications may reduce the capsular volume.

5. Limit shoulder motion until after the MR imaging to avoid physiologic extravasation on redressing; leave the patient in a gown.

6. If multiple intra-articular injections are anticipated in a single day (irrespective of specific joint), consider preparing a single-day, multidose saline bag, such as 0.4 mL of gadolinium in a 100-mL sterile saline infusion bag.

For those with less experience with articular injections and for those in an academic institution with learners participating, separation of contrast agents may be of benefit to prohibit accidental infusion of gadolinium into the bursa, potentially confounding MR interpretation. For the experienced arthrographer with a high frequency of correct needle placement, iodinated and gadolinium contrast agents can be mixed,[9] allowing fluoroscopic confirmation and MR infusion without needle/tubing manipulation.

Gadolinium diluted 1:125: 8 mL

Lidocaine 1%: 3 mL

Iodinated contrast, 300 mg/L: 3 mL

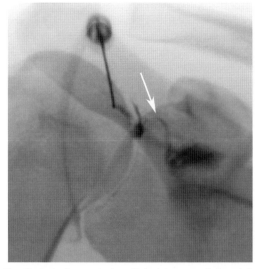

Fig. 2. Anterior-posterior digital image of the right shoulder shows the position of the injection needle via the rotator cuff interval, with the tip abutting the superior medial margin of the humeral head. Injected contrast (*arrow*) flows briskly toward the subcoracoid recess.

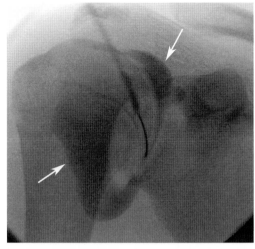

Fig. 4. Anterior-posterior digital image of the right shoulder shows correct positioning of the injection needle at the inferior articular space with ready opacification of the glenohumeral capsule (*arrows*).

this approach can be valuable for an MR facility separated from a fluoroscopy suite. The patient may be seated in a chair for this injection with the humerus internally rotated, forearm resting on the lap. Alternatively, the patient is positioned prone on the fluoroscopy table. The posterolateral margin of the acromion is palpated and marked. The arthrographer also palpates the coracoid. Using a 38-mm (1-5-inch) 22G spinal needle and the usual sterile technique, the needle is inserted

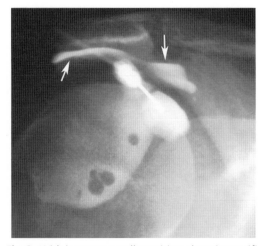

Fig. 3. With incorrect needle position, there is opacification of the subacromial bursa (*arrows*), without intra-articular contrast.

approximately 2 to 3 cm inferior to the acromial mark, with the tip oriented to project toward the coracoid. The needle is advanced until the humeral head is encountered.[12] A test injection of lidocaine 1% can used to assess the ease of the injection, with a correctly positioned needle allowing free infusion of solution with no pain for the patient. If fluoroscopy is available, a test injection with iodinated contrast is used to confirm the intra-articular needle position. The gadolinium contrast can then be infused at a concentration similar to the rotator cuff interval approach.

Most sports medicine physicians appreciate completion of a challenge test at the time of joint injection by including anesthetic into the distending fluids. Besides potentially resulting in a more comfortable examination, a preinjection and postinjection pain scale can be acquired with the outcome recorded in the procedural report. Theoretically, an improvement in pain after intra-articular injection of anesthetic supports the concept that some degree of internal derangement contributes to the patient's symptoms. The challenge is imperfect because some patients may not report accurate scales. In addition, results may be confounded by symptoms induced by the capsular distention or by shoulder or emotional confinement within the bore of the magnet.

MR Sequences

Selection of optimum protocols depends primarily on the choice of contrast agent. Typically, if

Problem Solving

- Contrast allergy:

  ○ Gadolinium contrast: saline can be used as the distending agent, with appropriate modification of the MR imaging protocol by emphasizing T2-weighted sequences (especially with fat saturation) and eliminating fat-suppressed T1-weighted imaging.

  ○ Iodinated contrast: there are several alternatives to consider, taking into account the arthrographer's experience, patient preference, and imaging center support. The risk of true allergic reaction including urticaria and respiratory distress is extremely low[11] but not nonexistent. Furthermore, any coincident complaints or reactions may be incorrectly associated with the procedure. Therefore, some advocate full steroid preparation before the procedure if iodinated contrast is used. For the highly experienced arthrographer, the injection can be completed using the traditional method, with the exception of infusion of lidocaine instead of iodinated contrast to test needle position. If the needle is fully intracapsular, infusion will be uninhibited manually and will not cause patient discomfort. Another problem-solving tool is the use of ultrasonographic guidance for the injection, should this imaging modality be available. Ultrasonography provides direct visualization of needle placement and subsequent capsular distention, precluding the need for fluoroscopic inspection. Some imagers may also advocate the use of indirect arthrography for these cases.

Procedural Risks

- Infection: with appropriate attention to sterile technique for preparation of the procedural tray and for the procedure activity, the risk of infection is exceedingly low at approximately 1 in 25,000.[11] All vials of solution should be inspected for expiration date and intact lids/seals.

- Bleeding: routine procedural precautions should be observed including discontinuing any anticoagulation medication before the procedure if possible, and application of manual pressure for postprocedural hemostasis. Many arthrographers do not require discontinuation of low-dose (82.5 mg) daily aspirin therapy. Laboratory evaluation of bleeding parameters is not indicated given the relatively low invasiveness of the procedure, although these tests could be obtained in high-risk patients if there is a question. Because this is considered an invasive elective procedure and because there are other noninvasive techniques as well as alternative imaging modalities, such as ultrasonography, injection should not be completed in the setting of full anticoagulation.

gadolinium is used, T1-weighted fat-saturated techniques and T2-weighted techniques are often used.

Coronal planes tend to be emphasized for viewing the supraspinatus tendon and superior labral biceps complex, including T1-weighted fat-saturated, proton density, and T2-weighted sequences. Sagittal sequences, T2-weighted or T1-weighted fat-saturated, are helpful to evaluate atrophy of the muscles of the rotator cuff and paralabral cysts. Axial planes, especially proton density and T1-weighted fat-saturated, are critical for evaluating the anterior inferior and posterior labrum. Some imagers advocate imaging in the abducted, external rotation (ABER) position to allow improved visualization of the undersurface of the supraspinatus tendon (oblique coronal) or the anterior inferior labrum (oblique axial).

ELBOW

Triceps and biceps injuries are common athletic injuries, and MR arthrography is not needed to diagnose these injuries. However, articular distention is especially valuable for evaluation of articular surfaces and supporting ligamentous structures, especially in the athlete. Elbow injuries in athletes most commonly involve overhand sports in which there is repeated valgus stress. Medial tension-lateral compression in the valgus position may lead to injuries of the ulnar collateral ligament (UCL), flexor-pronator tendon complex, ulnar neuropathy, osteochondritis dissecans (OCD) (especially of the capitellum), and loose bodies. MR arthrography provides enhanced evaluation of many of these injuries including UCL partial or complete tears, OCD of the capitellum, and differentiation of loose bodies from synovial proliferation.[13]

UCL injuries are most commonly seen in sports with repetitive overhead throwing such as football, baseball, tennis, and the javelin throw due to valgus stress with the elbow flexed.[14,15] The phases of the throwing cycle placing the greatest stress on the UCL are the late-cocking and acceleration phases.[16] Clinical diagnosis of UCL tear, especially a partial tear that limits function/ strength but does not show frank instability on examination using a milking sign, is difficult, warranting advanced imaging for anatomic inspection. MR arthrography is superior to MR imaging for detection of partial tears of the UCL. A study by Timmerman and colleagues[17] showed MRI sensitivity of 57% for partial thickness tears of the anterior band UCL. In contrast, Schwartz and colleagues[18] showed a sensitivity of 92% for MR arthrography for detecting partial tears of the same component of the UCL.

OCD of the capitellum is a common cause of lateral elbow pain and loose bodies in adolescent athletes. The injury is probably the result of repetitive lateral impaction and compressive forces on the lateral joint during throwing activities.[19] Routine MR imaging provides a noninvasive sensitive tool for evaluation of subchondral marrow abnormalities including OCD. However, this technique provides only limited evaluation of the integrity of the overlying cartilage and the stability of the devascularized fragment(s).[20] Indirect MR arthrography is a useful tool, providing a noninvasive assessment of the fragment/host interface for granulation tissue and viability of the fragment. However, MR arthrography provides superior assessment of articular cartilage integrity and potential isolation of the fragment.[20]

MR arthrography can also be used to distinguish intracapsular loose bodies from synovial nodules and plica.[21] Large loose bodies may be readily detectable on routine MR imaging. MR arthrography, however, provides more precise delineation of intracapsular versus extracapsular calcifications.[22]

There are 2 commonly used approaches for elbow joint injection: lateral radiocapitellar and posterolateral marginal to the triceps tendon. A less common technique, the posterior transtriceps approach, may also be used. The direct lateral approach is more simplistic with a high degree of success on the first attempt. However, this approach is contraindicated when evaluating for lateral pain because local anesthetic infiltration or any iatrogenic contrast extravasation may confuse the imaging picture.

Technique

Lateral radiocapitellar approach
Preparatory materials
Gadolinium diluted 1:250: 9 mL
Lidocaine 1%: 3 mL
Iodinated contrast, 300 mg/L: <5 mL
Lidocaine 1%: local anesthesia
21G butterfly needle

Before positioning for the actual procedure, the elbow is extended and the lateral dimple localized.

The examiner's index finger is positioned at the most volar margin of the dimple, and the patient's forearm is rotated from prone to supine with the elbow flexed 30°. The radial head is confirmed by motion under the examiner's finger. The skin is marked corresponding to the anterior margin of the lateral radiocapitellar joint line (a task to be completed before anesthetic infiltration as landmarks will be lost).[23] The patient is seated at the side of the fluoroscopy table, leaning in to the spot view of the imaging tube. The elbow is flexed 90°, oriented horizontal to the ground, thumb pointing upward (**Fig. 5**). Alternatively, the patient can be positioned prone on the table, with the affected arm overhead with similar elbow/forearm positioning.[23] Local infiltration with 1% lidocaine provides adequate anesthesia. With orientation perpendicular to the ground, observing sterile technique, a 21G butterfly needle is advanced into the lateral joint line. The butterfly needle is advantageous because the needle would infrequently be hubbed when in the proper position, allowing a rapid visual on needle positioning. A subtle pop is often noted by the arthrographer as the needle penetrates the taught capsule. Less than 1 mL of iodinated contrast is infused under fluoroscopic observation for confirmation of the intra-articular position. Usually, the intra-articular contrast flows briskly into the anterior capsular recess (**Fig. 6**). Subsequently, 12 mL of the gadolinium solution are infused for adequate capsular distention.

Posterolateral paratriceps tendon
This approach is the technique of choice for cases where lateral joint line symptomatology is under

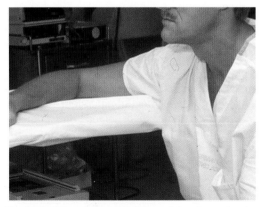

Fig. 5. For the radiocapitellar or lateral paratendon approach for elbow arthrography, the patient can be seated at the side of the table with the arm parallel to the table, lateral side up. The elbow is flexed 90°. For optimum position, the hand is perpendicular to the table.

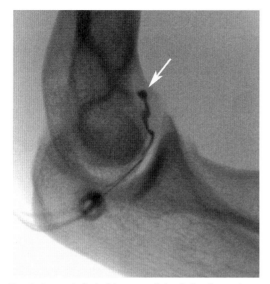

Fig. 6. Lateral digital image of the left elbow shows correct positioning of the needle at the radiocapitellar joint. Injected contrast (*arrow*) flows briskly into the anterior capsular recess.

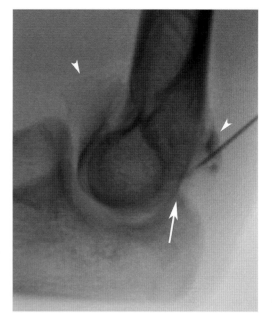

Fig. 7. Lateral digital image of the right elbow shows positioning of a needle at the posterolateral elbow with appropriate obliquity to pass superior to the olecranon process (*arrow*) to the olecranon fossa and finally the joint capsule. Contrast opacifies the joint capsule (*arrowheads*).

evaluation. Although the joint line may be accessible from a medial paratendon approach, the ulnar nerve position makes this approach less desirable.

Positioning of the patient is similar to the lateral approach. With the elbow flexed 90°, the skin is marked approximately 2 cm above the palpable olecranon margin, at the lateral margin of the triceps tendon. With sterile technique, a 38-mm (1.5-inch) 22G spine needle is inserted at the skin mark and angled deep to the tip of the olecranon to the posterior humeral capsular margin in the olecranon fossa. Again, infusion of iodinated contrast confirms the intra-articular position, with contrast flowing into the anterior capsular recess (**Fig. 7**).

Posterior transtriceps Although not as commonly used, this posterior approach can be used when the lateral joint line is the area of interest. For the technique described by Lohman and colleagues,[24] the patient is prone or supine on the table with the arm positioned horizontally. Similar to the techniques described earlier, the elbow is flexed approximately 90°. A posterior point midline between the epicondyles just above the olecranon is marked. Under sterile technique after local anesthesia, the injection needle is advanced with slight cephalad orientation until

---

Tips and Tricks

1. A true lateral projection for fluoroscopy facilitates anatomic orientation and expedites needle repositioning for all approaches.

2. For the posterolateral approach, the steepness of needle orientation and overall depth of penetration are often greater than expected. If the injection needle encounters bone at a depth of 1 or 1.5 cm, the needle is likely encountering the olecranon tip, extracapsular.

3. The decision whether to seat the patient at the side of the fluoroscopy table should be considered at the initial patient encounter. Patients with excessive anxiety or with a history/potential for adverse reaction to the concept of a procedure with needles (such as vasovagal events) should be examined supine on the table rather than seated at the side of the table.

Procedural Risks

Identical to those for shoulder injection.

the posterior humeral cortex is reached. A test injection of iodinated contrast should show contrast flowing rapidly away from the needle tip, opacifying the capsule.

MR Sequences

If the goal of MR interrogation is to determine the integrity of collateral ligaments, coronal planes of imaging are emphasized, especially those that are water sensitive (T2 and T2*) and T1-weighted sequences sensitive to gadolinium products, especially with fat saturation, to increase conspicuity of extra-articular or intrasubstance fluid collection. High-resolution proton density images, with or without fat saturation, provide an excellent profile of ligaments. Axial imaging provides a supplemental plane of investigation. In contrast, because osteochondral lesions most commonly occur at the capitellum, sagittal plane imaging is critical for this diagnosis. Again, T2-weighted and T1-weighted fat-suppressed imaging is key for diagnosing OCD lesions. Coronal plane imaging provides an alternative plane profile important for further assessment.

WRIST

Injuries of the wrist are common in athletes, including ligamentous and cartilaginous injuries. Triangular fibrocartilage complex (TFC) tears may be caused by traumatic injuries such as falls or by overuse injury, commonly associated with gymnastics, racket sports, and golf.[25,26] Injury of the scapholunate ligament can occur from excessive extension and ulnar deviation, such as a fall on an outstretched hand.[27] Contact sports account for many of these injuries. Tears of the lunatotriquetral ligaments are much less common than scapholunate ligament tears but also occur from a fall on an outstretched hand.[27]

Routine arthrography of the wrist has largely fallen by the wayside since the introduction of MR imaging. With appropriate attention to technique, 1.5-T and 3-T MR imaging of the wrist is diagnostic for evaluation of common sources of intrinsic and extrinsic pathologic conditions in athletes including occult fracture and lunate avascular necrosis. Injuries of the intrinsic ligaments and lunate chondromalacia (±ulnar positive variance) can frequently be detected as well.[28] However, more subtle conditions including delaminating cartilage injuries and partial tears of intrinsic ligaments (especially the triangular fibrocartilage) are better seen on MR arthrography. Several studies have shown that MR arthrography of the wrist has excellent accuracy for diagnosing tears of the intrinsic ligaments,[29] perhaps almost

equivalent to arthroscopy for the diagnosis of intrinsic ligament tear and cartilage lesions.[30]

Technique

Most imagers consider a unicompartmental injection satisfactory for the diagnosis of most injuries of intrinsic ligaments while limiting the patient symptomatology that frequently accompanies wrist injections. Thus, a diagnostic examination without problematic patient motion can usually be obtained.

Unicompartmental, radiocarpal
Preparatory materials
    Gadolinium diluted 1:250: 4 mL
    Lidocaine 1%: 2 mL
    Iodinated contrast, 300 mg/L: <5 mL
    Lidocaine 1%: local anesthesia
    21G butterfly needle

The patient is supine on the table, arm resting comfortably at the side. A small towel is placed on the table under the radiocarpal joint to accommodate the typical volar orientation of the joint, allowing a perpendicular approach for the injection (**Fig. 8**). A point at the perimeter of the radial-scaphoid joint is marked using fluoroscopy (**Fig. 9**).[31,32] Following sterile precautions, a 21G butterfly needle is directed perpendicularly into the radiocarpal joint with the expectation of a pop as the dorsal capsule is entered. Contrast is used for confirmation of articular position, with rapid migration of the contrast either into the volar radiocarpal recess at the radial margin or coursing along the articular space toward the ulnar margin (**Fig. 10**). There is considerable variability in capsular volume at the radiocarpal joint and ultimately, the amount of solution infused depends on patient symptomatology and intrinsic ligament integrity. Approximately 3 mL of a 2:1 solution of

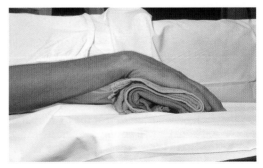

Fig. 8. For injection of the radiocarpal joint space, the patient is positioned supine with the arm fully extended at the side, palm down. A small towel is placed under the wrist for approximately 20° flexion.

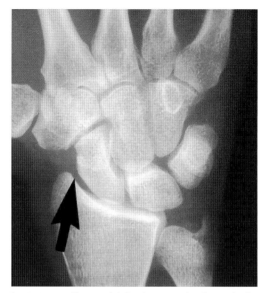

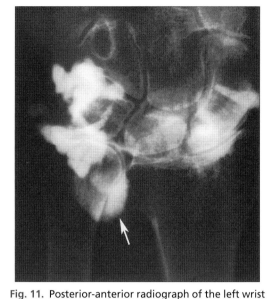

Fig. 9. For radiocarpal injection, a point is marked at the radial perimeter of the joint line (*arrow*). With a perpendicular approach, a butterfly needle is properly placed for radiocarpal articular opacification.

Fig. 11. Posterior-anterior radiograph of the left wrist after radiocarpal injection shows abnormal opacification of the distal radioulnar joint capsule (*arrow*) indicating a TFC ligament tear.

dilute gadolinium and 1% lidocaine are infused. The patient will typically note a sensation of increasing pressure coincident with the examiner noting increasing tension behind the injection. In the circumstance that there is a tear of 1 of the 3 intrinsic ligaments of the wrist (scapholunate, lunate-triquetral, or TFC), contrast passes into neighboring compartments allowing an increased volume of contrast solution to be injected, often up to 4.5 mL (**Fig. 11**). Intermittent

fluoroscopic observation is helpful to identify the contrast migration and estimate ultimate contrast volume. It is important to gauge the symptoms and the tension of the injection to avoid overdistention. If too much discomfort is induced, involuntary motion renders the MR examination nondiagnostic.

Tricompartmental

If a 3-comparment injection is chosen, most arthrographers begin with the radiocarpal joint as discussed earlier because ligament injury results in multicompartment opacification, obviating the need for separate injections at the midcarpal and/or distal radioulnar joints.[32,33]

After the radiocarpal injection, a midcarpal injection can be completed. The folded towel under the wrist is removed. A 21G butterfly needle is most easily passed into the midcarpal joint space at the quadrilateral space demarcated by the capitate, hamate, lunate, and triquetrum (**Fig. 12**).[33] Similar to the radiocarpal space, a pop is frequently sensed on needle tip entry. The volume for this joint capsule is approximately 2.5 mL.

The distal radioulnar joint is the easiest of the 3 injections. With the hand positioned palm down on the table, a butterfly needle is passed directly to the distal/radial margin of the ulnar head (**Fig. 13**).[34] Similar to the glenohumeral capsule, redundancy over the ulnar head allows placement of the needle at a bone margin covered by

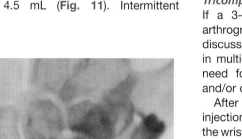

Fig. 10. Digital posterior-anterior image after contrast infusion into the radiocarpal joint capsule shows contrast profiling the articular cartilage and distending the multiple marginal recesses (*arrows*).

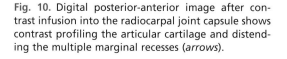

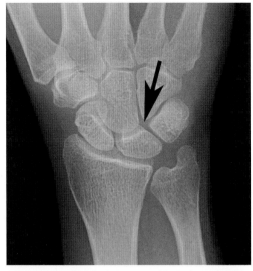

Fig. 12. For midcarpal injection, a mark is placed at the juncture of the capitate, lunate, hamate, and triquetrum (*arrow*). A butterfly needle can be advanced perpendicular to this mark for confident intraarticular placement.

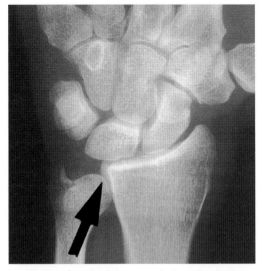

Fig. 13. Because the joint capsule is redundant over the ulnar head, the distal radioulnar capsule can be accessed by advancing a needle directly to the bone margin at the distal radial margin of the ulnar head (*arrow*).

capsule rather than a narrow articular space, facilitating capsular entry. Although a needle can be placed at the most proximal margin of the distal radioulnar interface hoping to engage the capsular margin, this technique requires patience and finesse and is not recommended. When accessed, this small joint accommodates about 1 to 1.5 mL of solution.

MR Sequences

MR arthrography has the most beneficial role in the assessment of integrity of the intrinsic ligaments and chondral lesions of the lunate, compared with routine MR imaging. Therefore, coronal plane imaging is key for evaluation. Again, water-sensitive as well as gadolinium-sensitive sequences are the most beneficial. For intrinsic

ligaments, high-resolution proton density imaging is also helpful. Axial plane imaging is probably the most useful secondary plane, although sagittal projections also play an important role for evaluating lunate chondromalacia.

MR arthrography is an accepted method of interrogation of joints of the upper extremities for injury and derangement. Although not indicated for all patients and all clinical scenarios, capsular distention can aid visualization of subtle intracapsular structures. In particular, incomplete injuries with few associated secondary imaging signs of injury may also be delineated to better advantage than with traditional MR imaging. With appropriate patient selection and attention to proper technique, MR arthrography can be completed with little discomfort and extremely low risk to the patient.

Tips and Tricks:

1. The wrist palmar flexion for the radiocarpal injection facilitates correct capsular positioning and thus decreases procedural discomfort for the patient.

2. Although adequate distention is desirable, distention to the point of frank pain usually results in suboptimal MR because of patient motion, voluntary or involuntary. Intermittent fluoroscopic observation as well as sensitivity to ongoing patient expressions and gestures provide insight about capsular tension.

Procedural Risks

Identical to those for shoulder injection.

REFERENCES

1. Oh DK, Yoon YC, Kwon JW, et al. Comparison of indirect isotropic MR arthrography and conventional MR arthrography of labral lesions and rotator cuff tears: a prospective study. AJR Am J Roentgenol 2009;192:473–9.

2. Magee T, Williams D, Mani N. Shoulder MR arthrography: which patient group benefits the most? AJR Am J Roentgenol 2004;183:969–74.

3. Guanche CA, Jones DC. Clinical testing for tears of the glenoid labrum. Arthroscopy 2003;19(5):517–23.

4. Holtby R, Razmjour H. Accuracy of the Speed's and Yergason's tests in detecting biceps pathology and SLAP lesions: comparison with arthroscopic findings. Arthroscopy 2004;20(23):231–6.

5. Rafii M, Firooznia O, Minkoff J, et al. Rotator cuff lesions: signal patterns at MR imaging. Radiology 1990;177:817–23.

6. Palmer WE, Brown JH, Rosenthal DI. Rotator cuff: evaluation with fat-suppressed MR arthrography. Radiology 1993;188:683–7.

7. Duc SR, Mengiardi B, Pfirrmann CW, et al. Diagnostic performance of MR arthrography after rotator cuff repair. AJR Am J Roentgenol 2006;186:237–41.

8. Jacobson JA, Lin J, Jamada DA, et al. Aids to successful shoulder arthrography performed with a fluoroscopically guided anterior approach. Radiographics 2003;23:373–8.

9. Brown RR, Clarke DW, Daffner RH. Is a mixture of gadolinium and iodinated contrast material safe during MR arthrography? AJR Am J Roentgenol 2000;175:1087.

10. Kaye J, Freiberger R. Positive contrast shoulder arthrography. In: Freiberger RH, Kaye JJ, editors. Arthrography. New York: Appleton-Century-Crofts; 1979. p. 137–64.

11. Farmer KD, Highes PM. Fluoroscopically guided technique using a posterior approach. AJR Am J Roentgenol 2002;178:433–4.

12. Yellin J, Peterson JJ. MR arthrography. Appl Radiol 2010;39. Available at: http://www.appliedradiology.com/Issues/2010/09/Articles/AR_09-10_Peterson/MR-arthrography.aspx. Accessed April 4, 2012.

13. Dodd M. Tommy John surgery: pitcher's best friend. USA Today 2003;11. Available at: http://www.usatoday.com/sports/baseball/2003-07-28-cover-tommy-john_x.htm. Accessed April 1, 2012.

14. Petty DH, Andrews JR, Fleisig GS, et al. Ulnar collateral ligament reconstruction in high school baseball players: clinical results and injury risk factors. Am J Sports Med 2004;32:1158–64.

15. Hang Y, Lippert F, Spolek G, et al. Biomechanical study of the pitching elbow. Int Orthop 1979;3:217–23.

16. Timmerman LA, Schwartz ML, Andrews JR. Preoperative evaluation of the ulnar collateral ligament by magnetic resonance imaging and computed tomography arthrography: evaluation in 25 baseball players with surgical confirmation. Am J Sports Med 1994;22:26–32.

17. Schwartz ML, al-Zahrani S, Morwessel RM, et al. Ulnar collateral ligament injury in the throwing athlete: evaluation of saline enhanced MR arthrography. Radiology 1995;197:297–9.

18. Pappas AM. Osteochondrosis dissecans. Clin Orthop Relat Res 1981;158:59–69.

19. Ouellette H, Bredella M, Labis J, et al. MR imaging of the elbow in baseball pitchers. Skeletal Radiol 2008; 37:115–21.

20. Awaya H, Schweitzer ME, Feng SA, et al. Elbow synovial fold syndrome: MR imaging findings. Am J Roentgenol 2001;177:1377–81.

21. Steinbach L, Schwartz M. Elbow arthrography. Radiol Clin North Am 1998;36:635–49.

22. Hudson TM. The elbow. In: Freiberger RH, Kaye JJ, editors. Arthrography. New York: Appleton-Century-Crofts; 1979. p. 261–76.

23. Morrey BF, Berquist TH. The elbow. In: Berquist TH, editor. Imaging of orthopedic trauma. New York: Raven; 1992. p. 675–700.

24. Lohman M, Borrero C, Casagranda B, et al. The posterior transtriceps approach for elbow arthrography: a forgotten approach? Skeletal Radiol 2009;38: 513–6.

25. Palmer AK, Werner FW. The triangular fibrocartilage complex of the wrist: anatomy and function. J Hand Surg Am 1981;6:153–62.

26. Mayfield JK, Johnson RP, Kilcoyne RK. Carpal dislocations: pathomechanics and progressive perilunar instability. J Hand Surg Am 1980;5:226–41.

27. Dobyns JH, Linscheid RL, Chao EY, et al. Traumatic instability of the wrist. Instr Course Lect 1975;24: 182–99.

28. Schmitt R, Christopoulos G, Meier R, et al. Direct MR arthrography of the wrist in comparison with arthroscopy: a prospective study on 125 patients. Rofo 2003;175:911–9 [in German].

29. Scheck RJ, Romagnolo A, Hiemer R, et al. The carpal ligaments in MR arthrography of the wrist: correlation with standard MRI and wrist arthroscopy. J Magn Reson Imaging 1999;9:464–74.

30. Gilula LA, Totty WG, Week PM. Wrist arthrography. Radiology 1983;146:555–6.

31. Wood MB, Berquist TH. The hand and wrist. In: Berquist TH, editor. Imaging of orthopedic trauma. New York: Raven; 1992. p. 749–96.

32. Levinsohn EM, Palmer AK, Coren AB, et al. Wrist arthrography: the value of the three compartment injection technique. Skeletal Radiol 1987;16(7):539–44.

33. Dalinka MK, Melvin LT, Osterman AL, et al. Wrist arthrography. Radiol Clin North Am 1981;19: 217–26.

34. Lomasney LM, Cooper R. Simplification of distal radioulnar joint injection. Radiology 1996;199:278–9.

Conventional Radiographic Evaluation of Athletic Injuries to the Hand

Narayan Sundaram, MD, MBA[a],*, Jacob Bosley, MD[b],
Gregory Scott Stacy, MD[a]

KEYWORDS

- Athletic • Sports • Hand • Finger • Fractures • Dislocations • Management • Radiographs

KEY POINTS

- Athletic injuries to the hand are common and encompass a diverse spectrum of injuries.
- Radiographs represent the most appropriate imaging modality for the initial evaluation of most hand injuries, although advanced imaging modalities, such as magnetic resonance imaging and ultrasonography, are useful in certain circumstances.
- A basic understanding of the clinical management of athletic injuries of the hand will enhance the radiologist's ability to convey pertinent information to the referring clinician, including recommendation for orthopedic consultation.

INTRODUCTION

Athletic injuries to the hand are common and encompass a diverse spectrum of injuries. These injuries can include fractures, soft tissue injuries, or both. Athletic injuries to the hand can be due to a variety of mechanisms and can be seen in a variety of sports. Prompt attention and accurate diagnosis should be provided to patients with athletic injuries to the hand to allow for appropriate treatment and to prevent serious complications that may preclude further athletic activity. Conventional radiography is the most common imaging modality used for the diagnosis of athletic hand injuries, although advanced modalities such as computed tomography (CT), magnetic resonance imaging (MRI), or ultrasonography may be needed to diagnose the full extent of injury.

Athletic injuries are among the most common causes of hand fractures in young patients.[1,2] Most such fractures result from low-energy trauma, but nevertheless, can alter an athlete's performance and result in a loss of playing time. Radiographs can diagnose accurately various types of athletic hand fractures, which are presented in this article. This article also provides a brief description of the clinical management of selected injuries.

RADIOGRAPHY

Accurate diagnosis of athletic injuries to the hand depends on proper radiographic evaluation. Improper positioning or radiographic exposure factors may result in overlooked or invisible fractures, which in turn can result in debilitating complications.

Radiography of phalangeal injuries should consist of at least 3 projections: PA (posteroanterior), lateral, and externally rotated oblique views.[3] A step wedge can be used on the lateral view to separate the fingers and prevent overlap. An internally rotated oblique view may be added to the aforementioned 3 views to increase diagnostic

[a] Department of Radiology, The University of Chicago Medical Center, 5841 South Maryland Avenue, Chicago, IL 60637, USA; [b] Section of Orthopaedic Surgery and Rehabilitation, Department of Surgery, The University of Chicago Medical Center, 5841 South Maryland Avenue, Chicago, IL 60637, USA
* Corresponding author.
E-mail address: nsundaram@radiology.bsd.uchicago.edu

Radiol Clin N Am 51 (2013) 239–255
http://dx.doi.org/10.1016/j.rcl.2012.09.015
0033-8389/13/$ – see front matter © 2013 Published by Elsevier Inc.

confidence for phalangeal fractures. Some practices include a PA view of the entire hand rather than limiting the projection to the injured finger.[3]

For suspected metacarpal fracture or dislocation, PA, lateral, and semipronated oblique views of the hand are recommended for initial evaluation. A supinated oblique view of the hand can be considered for visualization of the base of the fifth metacarpal and the fifth carpometacarpal joint.

Three views of the thumb are appropriate for suspected thumb fracture or dislocation and include a lateral view, an oblique view, and either a PA or an anteroposterior (AP) view. The PA view of the thumb is obtained by having the patient rest his or her thumb on a sponge support block that is placed on the image receptor. Although the PA technique may result in some loss of bone definition because of the increased object-to-image receptor distance, positioning for this view is generally easier for the patient than the hyperpronation necessary for the AP view. Stress views of the thumb in the setting of a suspected ulnar collateral ligament injury are controversial and are discussed later.

At our institution, radiographs are obtained after the patient has removed all jewelry, if possible. For the average-sized patient, radiographs of the hands and fingers can be performed with a peak kilovolt of 50 to 60, milliamperes of 1 to 3, at a distance of 40 in, without the use of a grid. Finally, the radiologist should be informed of the patient's clinical history and any specific questions of the referring clinician to ensure an accurate and specific diagnosis.

PHALANGEAL AND INTERPHALANGEAL JOINT INJURIES

The finger consists of the proximal phalanx (P1), the middle phalanx (P2), the distal phalanx (P3), the interphalangeal joints, and the surrounding soft tissues. The authors recommend designating the digits of the hand as the thumb, the index finger, the middle finger, the ring finger, and the fifth finger; labeling the fingers numerically can result in confusion, particularly when ordering radiographs (eg, the "third finger" may be interpreted to represent either the middle finger, if including the thumb in the numbering scheme, or the ring finger, if not including the thumb).

Distal Phalangeal Injuries

Of the bones of the fingers, the distal phalanges are the most commonly fractured.[4] The middle finger is most commonly affected, followed by the thumb.[2] Distal phalangeal injuries are most often due to crush injuries or direct blow

mechanisms and may be associated with significant soft tissue injuries involving the fingertip and/or nail bed (eg, a soccer player wearing cleated shoes steps on the finger of another player). Fracture patterns described with crush injuries include longitudinal, transverse, and comminuted ("crushed eggshell"). Distal phalangeal fractures are often stabilized by the nail plate dorsally as well as by fibrous septae that extend from the bone to the skin volarly and minimize displacement of fracture fragments. The volar fibrous septae, however, form closed compartments that cause severe pain when expanded by edema and hematoma. Comminuted and longitudinal fractures tend to result in fragments that remain in anatomic alignment, whereas transverse fractures are often associated with volar or dorsal displacement that may warrant orthopedic referral (**Fig. 1**). Displaced fractures are often associated with nail bed injuries, and the nail bed can occasionally become interposed between fracture fragments, preventing reduction[5]; therefore, the radiologist should report any widening of the fracture line on the lateral view, as this could indicate entrapment of the nail bed. Axial loading injuries, not uncommon in baseball, football, and karate, may also cause longitudinal or transverse fractures; fractures that extend through the base of the phalanx to the distal interphalangeal (DIP) joint must be reported, as they may result in displacement and instability, warranting surgical referral.[2]

Intra-articular fractures of the base of the distal phalanx can also result from avulsion of either the extensor or the flexor tendon. The extensor tendon of the finger splits dorsal to the proximal phalanx to form a central slip, which inserts on the dorsal aspect of the base of the middle phalanx, and 2 additional lateral slips that receive fibers from the intrinsic muscles of the hand and combine distally as a terminal tendon to attach to the dorsal aspect of the base of the distal phalanx. "Mallet finger" (also known as "drop finger" or "baseball finger") refers to disruption of this terminal tendon at its insertion. Mallet finger occurs because of forceful flexion of an extended DIP joint, for example, when a ball strikes the tip of a finger. Additional, albeit less frequent, mechanisms of mallet finger include volar subluxation of the distal phalanx on the middle phalanx and direct trauma to the dorsal distal phalanx.[6] Clinically, mallet finger can present as a flexion deformity of the DIP joint because of the action of the distal attachment of the uninjured flexor digitorum profundus tendon volarly. In most instances, mallet finger is associated with disruption of the distal extensor tendon without a fracture line evident on radiographs; in the acute setting, the patient

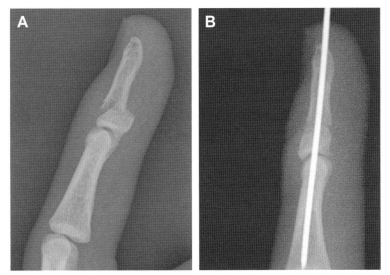

Fig. 1. A 20-year-old man who presents for care following a football injury to his middle finger. (A) Lateral radiograph shows a transverse fracture through the base of the distal phalanx with dorsal displacement of the distal fracture fragment that warranted surgical intervention in this patient. (B) Intraoperative fluoroscopy image shows pin fixation of the fracture.

is often able to extend the DIP joint, which may obscure a flexion deformity on radiographs. However, a "mallet fracture" can be diagnosed on radiographs when an avulsion fracture of the dorsal aspect of the base of the distal phalanx is evident (Fig. 2). If the avulsion fracture fragment involves more than 30% to 40% of the articular surface, if the fracture fragment is displaced by over 2 mm, or if there is volar displacement of the distal phalanx, surgical consultation is recommended.[7] Furthermore, the presence of a large avulsion fragment suggests additional injury to the ulnar and radial collateral ligaments (RCLs) of the DIP joint.[7] Mallet thumb (avulsion of the extensor pollicis longus) represents only 2% to 3% of all mallet injuries.[8]

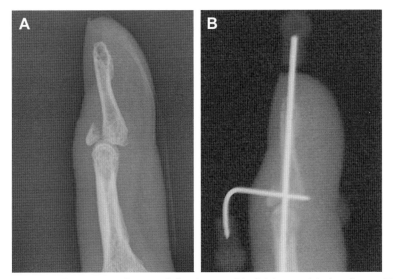

Fig. 2. A 33-year-old man who presents for care following a softball injury to his ring finger. (A) Lateral radiograph shows a mallet fracture (extensor tendon avulsion fracture) through the dorsal aspect of the base of the distal phalanx, warranting surgical intervention based on the size of the avulsed fragment as well as the volar subluxation of the distal phalanx relative to the middle phalanx. (B) Intraoperative fluoroscopy image shows pin fixation of the fracture and joint.

Clinically, closed fractures of the distal phalanx acutely require applying some type of immobilization to the DIP joint. This immobilization can be achieved with several different types of finger splints, including a Stack splint, a carefully molded alumafoam splint, a thermoplastic splint, or one of several commercially available splints. The goal of these splints is to immobilize the DIP joint in slight hyperextension, helping to bring the common extensor tendon or the avulsed piece of the distal phalanx into close approximation with the rest of the distal phalanx where it originated. It is important when immobilizing the DIP joint that patients retain full range of motion of their proximal interphalangeal joint (PIP) joint and are encouraged to keep moving the PIP joint to prevent stiffness. In additional, patients should be told that their DIP joint must be kept in a hyperextended position at all times to help the healing process and should be followed by a hand surgeon. Many physicians will advocate the use of rotating splints to allow for protection of the skin about the DIP joint.

Injury to the flexor digitorum profundus (FDP) tendon at the DIP joint occurs most commonly at the ring finger.[7] The flexor apparatus of the fingers consists of the FDP and the flexor digitorum superficialis (FDS) tendons, which are kept in close proximity to the proximal and middle phalanges by the flexor annular pulleys (fibrous bands) that are better imaged using MRI. At the level of the metacarpophalangeal (MCP) joint, the FDS splits and then rejoins at the level of the PIP, ultimately inserting onto the volar aspect of the middiaphysis of the middle phalanx. The FDP tendon runs between the split fibers of the FDS tendon and inserts on the volar aspect of the distal phalanx. Injury to the FDP tendon (termed "jersey finger" or "sweater finger") occurs when a finger is forcefully extended during active flexion, such as when an athlete grabs a moving player's jersey. Radiographs often can be normal with jersey finger, but avulsion fractures can be seen along the volar aspect of the base of the distal phalanx.[9] Smaller avulsed bony fragments can be seen volar to the middle or even proximal phalanx, indicating retraction of the FDP tendon (Fig. 3). Even with normal radiographs, if jersey finger is suspected clinically, patients should be referred to a hand surgeon for reattachment of the FDP.

Jersey finger is a frequently missed injury, especially if the FDP tendon is avulsed without a bony fragment. If the tendon avulses without a bony fragment, it may retract within the flexor sheath to the PIP joint or even retract all the way into the palm. Sometimes a lump can be palpated within the palm or along the course of the flexor sheath, which represents the avulsed tendon.

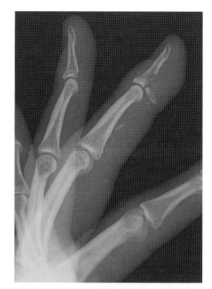

Fig. 3. A 32-year-old man who presents for care following a sports injury to his middle finger. Lateral radiograph shows a "jersey finger" consisting of a comminuted avulsion fracture of the volar aspect of the base of the distal phalanx, with smaller fracture fragments situated volar to the middle phalanx because of retraction by the flexor digitorum profundus tendon. The patient subsequently underwent surgical repair.

With an attached bony fragment, the tendon stump is typically held up at the A4 pulley and further retraction is prevented.[10] This method makes the tendon easier to find at the time of repair as well as prevents the blood supply to the tendon from being disrupted, which ultimately affects the rate of success for surgical repair of the tendon insertion. MRI or ultrasound may be used to confirm a suspected diagnosis of an FDP avulsion, as well as to help locate the tendon stump for the surgeon in anticipation of surgical repair. These injuries require early referral to a hand surgeon, as FDP tendons that have retracted into the palm should be repaired surgically within 3 weeks from the time of injury.[11] Treatment of chronic or missed jersey finger injuries can be considerably more complicated.

Distal Interphalangeal Joint Dislocation

The DIP joint is a ginglymus (hinge) joint surrounded by a capsuloligamentous complex.[12] Extension is constrained by the volar plate, a fibrocartilaginous structure that attaches to both phalanges along the palmar surface of the joint. Collateral ligaments provide radial and ulnar stability. Stability is enhanced by the adjacent insertions of the flexor and extensor tendons.[13,14] Owing to the stability of the joint as well as the short lever arm of the distal phalanx, dislocation of the DIP joint is an uncommon injury.[13] Patients usually present with obvious fingertip deformity; however, obtaining a fan lateral view of the hand or a lateral view of the injured finger is important, as DIP joint dislocation can be overlooked on PA and even oblique projections.

Simple dislocations of the DIP joint should be quickly reduced following diagnosis under digital or wrist block, followed by obtaining reduction radiographs afterward to confirm accurate reloca-tion of the joint. These injuries are commonly open, because of the minimal soft tissue coverage of the DIP joint, and any open wounds should be carefully inspected. Following successful reduction of the joint, the stability of the joint should be tested by passing the patient through a gentle range of motion. For dorsal dislocations, the patient should then be immobilized in a dorsal splint with the finger in approximately 20° of flexion. For volar disloca-tions, which are significantly less common than dorsal dislocations, the patient should be immobi-lized in full extension following successful reduction and managed in similar fashion as a mallet fracture. If closed reduction of a DIP dislocation cannot be completed, one should be suspicious for possible interposition of the proximal portion of the volar plate, although interposition of fracture fragments, a sesamoid bone, and flexor tendon have also been reported.[11] If the dislocation is truly irreduc-ible, the patient will need to be taken to the oper-ating room for open exploration and reduction.

Most fracture-dislocations of the DIP joint are palmar dislocations of the distal phalanx with fracture of the dorsal articular surface, which essentially represent large mallet injuries[15]; dorsal fracture-dislocations of the DIP joint occur infrequently.

Middle Phalangeal Fractures

Fractures of the middle phalanges are less common than those of the distal and proximal phalanges owing to the predominance of cortical bone and load-absorbing adjacent interphalangeal joints. Middle phalangeal fractures are usually caused by a direct blow or crush force perpendic-ular to the long axis of the middle phalanx, result-ing in a transverse or short oblique fracture. Angulation depends on the location of the fracture relative to the insertion of the FDS tendon along the volar aspect of the middle two-thirds of the bone. A fracture distal to the tendon attachment (distal third of the middle phalanx) results in volar apex angulation as the proximal fragment is flexed by the tendon; a fracture proximal to the tendon attachment (proximal third of the middle phalanx) results in dorsal apex angulation because of the volar pull of the distal fragment by the FDS as well as the extending force of the central slip of the extensor tendon on the proximal fragment.[2] Fracture of the mid diaphysis of the phalanx may be angulated in either direction or not angulated. Fracture fragment rotation must also be assessed, because the degree of rotation affects manage-ment. Indications for orthopedic referral include irreducible angulation or malrotation, oblique or spiral fractures (which are typically unstable), and intra-articular unicondylar or bicondylar fractures (**Fig. 4**).

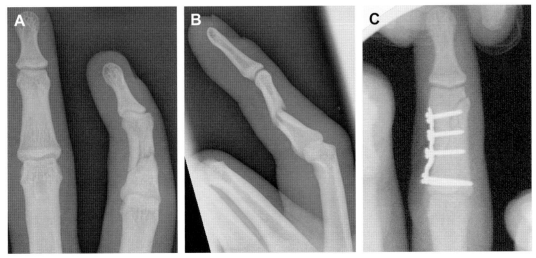

Fig. 4. A 17-year-old man who presents for care following a football injury to his ring finger. PA (*A*) and lateral (*B*) radiographs show a comminuted fracture of the middle phalanx with rotation and volar apex angulation that persisted despite attempted reduction, subsequently requiring surgical intervention. (*C*) Intraoperative fluoros-copy image shows plate and screw fixation of the fracture.

Volar Plate and Proximal Interphalangeal Joint Injuries

The PIP joint is the most commonly injured joint in sports.[8] Like the DIP joint, the PIP joint is a hinge joint that is stabilized by collateral ligaments and the fibrocartilaginous volar plate that connects the volar aspects of the proximal and middle phalanges across the PIP joint and prevents hyperextension. At the PIP joint, the volar plate is relatively thin and flexible at its proximal attachment, thickening at its distal attachment along the volar aspect of the base of the middle phalanx.[16] The plate attaches laterally to the accessory collateral ligaments. The collateral ligaments traverse the lateral and medial aspects of the joint and prevent ulnar and radial deviation.

Volar plate injuries occur because of hyperextension of the PIP joint, or because of rotational longitudinal compression. They can occur as isolated athletic injuries, particularly with ball-handling sports, or in combination with other injuries such as collateral ligament tears.[8] When avulsion of the volar plate occurs, it is usually at its distal attachment on the middle phalanx. Avulsions without bony fragments may show soft tissue swelling about the PIP joint or diffusely along the finger; further evaluation with MRI or sonography can be considered if clinical suspicion is high for a volar plate injury. An avulsion fracture is best seen on the lateral (or sometimes oblique) radiograph when a small piece of bone is seen volarly displaced from the base of the middle phalanx (**Fig. 5**). Injuries

resulting in a small fracture fragment and no joint subluxation can be treated conservatively. Larger fracture fragments (those involving greater than 30%–40% of the articular surface and to which the collateral ligaments remain attached) and joint subluxation (with widening of the dorsal aspect of the joint, implying injury to the dorsal capsule and at least 1 collateral ligament) are regarded as unstable and may necessitate surgical repair. If left untreated, patients with volar plate injuries can develop osteoarthritis, contractures, or joint laxity. A swan neck deformity may be evident, with hyperextension of the PIP joint and flexion of the DIP joint (**Fig. 6**). Alternatively, contractures can lead to a "pseudoboutonniere deformity," which is characterized by the inability of the patient to extend the injured finger[6]; this typically occurs if the volar plate is torn proximally,[8] and radiographs may reveal calcification in the area of the proximal volar plate.[16]

The extensor tendon central slip attaches distally onto a tubercle at the base of the middle phalanx. In the clinical setting of forced flexion of an extended PIP joint, this central slip can be avulsed. These injuries are common in basketball players and martial arts athletes. When the central slip of the extensor tendon is injured, extension at the PIP joint can be maintained by the lateral bands of the extensor tendon. However, if left untreated, the avulsed central slip will retract, and the lateral bands will sublux volarly, which results in a boutonniere deformity (flexion at the PIP joint and hyperextension at the DIP joint) (**Fig. 7**).[16] With this type of boutonniere deformity,

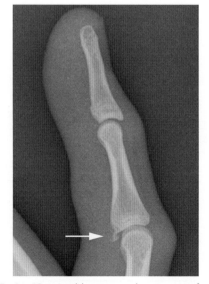

Fig. 5. An 18-year-old woman who presents for care following a volleyball injury to her 5th finger. Lateral radiograph shows a small volar plate avulsion fracture (*arrow*) that was treated conservatively.

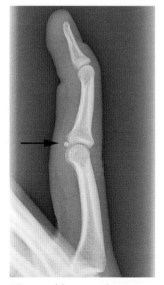

Fig. 6. An 19-year-old man who presents for care following a basketball injury to his fifth finger. Lateral radiograph shows a volar plate fracture fragment (*arrow*) and a swan neck deformity.

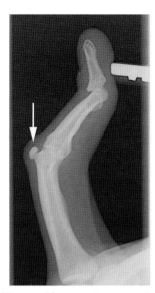

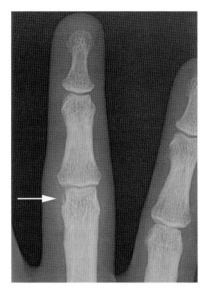

Fig. 7. A 22-year-old man who presents for care 6 months after sustaining a football injury to his fifth finger. Lateral radiograph shows an untreated extensor tendon central slip avulsion fracture (*arrow*) with resultant boutonniere deformity.

Fig. 8. A PA radiograph of the middle finger of a 38-year-old woman with pain following injury shows a small bone fragment (*arrow*) adjacent to the radial aspect of the head of the proximal phalanx, representing an avulsion fracture of the proximal attachment of the radial collateral ligament. The fracture was treated conservatively.

patients preserve their ability to extend the PIP joint passively (vs the aforementioned "pseudoboutonniere" deformity, with which patients cannot extend the PIP joint because of contracture). Central slip avulsions may or may not be associated with a fracture; if a fracture is present, it is best seen on the lateral view.

The proximal interphalangeal joint is stabilized along its ulnar and radial aspects by collateral ligaments that traverse the ulnar and radial sides of the joint. Collateral ligament injuries of the PIP joint are common. The mechanism of injury is usually due to axial loading and dorsiflexion forces with ulnar deviation at the joint; the proximal attachment of the RCL is most commonly injured with a partial tear.[8] Complete tears are rare and are usually associated with volar plate injuries (as mentioned earlier). On radiographs, collateral ligament injury can be suggested when there is greater than 10° of ulnar or radial angulation at an extended PIP joint[6] or soft tissue swelling about the ulnar or radial aspect of the PIP joint.[7] Repair is often recommended if the RCL of the index finger is involved.[8] Occasionally, a lateral avulsion fracture at the base of the middle phalanx or the head of the proximal phalanx may be evident (**Fig. 8**).[17] Large or displaced fractures warrant orthopedic referral.

PIP joint dislocation ("coach's finger") is common in sports, particularly in football, basketball, and baseball. Dorsal dislocation (of the middle phalanx) is the most frequent type of dislocation, occurring because of hyperextension with axial loading. It implies disruption of the volar plate (with or without avulsion fracture), both collateral ligaments, and the dorsal joint capsule. Lateral PIP joint dislocation, which also results in tearing of the volar plate and collateral ligaments, is less common.[16] Volar dislocation of the PIP joint is rare and may cause a tear of the central slip of the extensor tendon in addition to collateral ligament injury.[18]

As the deformity is usually obvious at the time of injury, reduction of dorsal PIP joint dislocations may be attempted without prior radiography; however, radiographs should be obtained after reduction to evaluate joint congruity.[18] Dorsal PIP joint dislocations may be irreducible if the volar plate becomes trapped within the joint. Furthermore, the head of the proximal phalanx may partially extend volarly between the volar plate and collateral ligament, or dorsally between the central and lateral slips of the extensor tendon, preventing adequate reduction. This partially extended head of the proximal phalanx is evident on lateral radiographs, which reveal that the middle and distal phalanges are oriented obliquely relative to the proximal phalanx.[7] Open repair may be recommended in such cases. Fracture-dislocations (most commonly dorsal dislocation of the middle phalanx with a volar lip fracture) should also be referred to an orthopedic surgeon (**Fig. 9**).[16]

Following reduction of a dorsal PIP joint dislocation, the patient should be passively taken through a range of motion to test their stability and reduction radiographs should be obtained afterward. The stability of the joint is best checked under fluoroscopy. By taking the patient through a gentle range of motion and making note of when the joint begins to sublux, treatment options are determined. Dorsal dislocations are most unstable in full extension. If the joint can be taken to 30° short of full extension with the joint still reduced and less than 20% of the articular surface is involved, the fracture is generally thought to be stable and is best treated conservatively with a dorsal blocking splint in 30° of flexion. In additional, passive range of motion under fluoroscopy can be analyzed to check if the joint is gliding appropriately or hinging through the fracture site.[19] Regardless of the direction of dislocation, reduction of PIP joint dislocation must be carefully scrutinized to determine the success of the reduction. The "V" sign, a radiolucent widening of the dorsal aspect of the PIP joint seen on the lateral view, is indicative of subtle joint instability. This joint instability is contrasted with the normal "C"-shape contour that exists between the proximal and middle phalanges. These injuries are notorious for being ignored initially, as well as progressing to

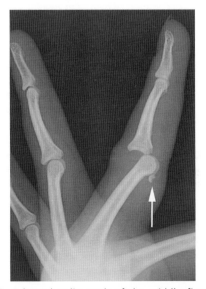

Fig. 9. A lateral radiograph of the middle finger of a 23-year-old woman with pain and deformity following injury shows dorsal dislocation at the proximal interphalangeal joint associated with a displaced volar plate avulsion fracture (*arrow*). Injuries such as these warrant orthopedic referral.

severe stiffness, sometimes even with appropriate treatment. Referral to a hand surgeon should occur shortly after diagnosis to ensure proper timing of any necessary surgical interventions as well as initiation of early range of motion exercises of the noninjured fingers.[15]

Proximal Phalanx Fractures

Proximal phalanx fractures in athletes are caused by a direct blow, hyperextension of the phalanx, or rotary force. The phalanx is in contact with the surrounding tendons, which can readily adhere to fractures resulting in tethering and limited motion. Unstable apex volar angulation is frequently a complication of these fractures, as the proximal fracture fragment is flexed by the intrinsic muscles while the distal fragment is extended by the central slip of the extensor tendon acting through the PIP joint.[2] The location and type of the fracture will determine the treatment, and careful evaluation of the PA, oblique and lateral views, is necessary to determine displacement, impaction, and angulation of fracture fragments. Fractures through the base of the proximal phalanx are usually transverse, with frequent volar apex angulation; a common pitfall of radiographic evaluation of these fractures is that fracture fragment angulation is often overlooked because of the superimposition of osseous structures on the lateral view.[2,7] Diaphyseal fractures may be transverse, oblique, or spiral. The adjacent tendon sheath and pulleys help to prevent displacement; however, oblique and spiral fractures are still susceptible to shortening, rotation, and instability, warranting orthopedic referral for potential fixation (**Fig. 10**).[2,7] Subcondylar fractures of the neck of the proximal phalanx also frequently result in rotation, and fixation is commonly necessary.[2] Intra-articular fractures involving the head of the proximal phalanx are usually unicondylar, but may be bicondylar or comminuted[8]; large displaced fragments are an indication for open reduction, internal fixation. Unlike the varied mechanisms of injury to other proximal phalanx fractures, thumb proximal phalanx fractures usually occur because of twisting injuries (for example, an equestrian rider's thumb getting stuck in the bridle).[7]

One of the most important concepts to address when dealing with middle and proximal phalanx fractures is the consequence of prolonged immobilization. The PIP joint is infamous for becoming severely stiff after any type of fracture of the finger. Initially, immobilization is often indicated, but the importance of appropriate follow-up and avoiding prolonged immobilization cannot be overstated. Studies have shown that immobilization of phalanx

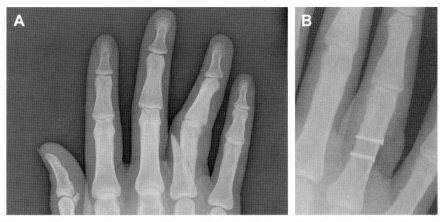

Fig. 10. A 24-year-old woman who presents for care following injury to her ring finger. PA radiograph (*A*) shows an unstable, long spiral-oblique fracture of the proximal phalanx. Note the resultant displacement, shortening, and rotational deformity, warranting surgical intervention in this patient. (*B*) Intraoperative fluoroscopy image shows screw fixation of the reduced fracture.

fractures for 4 weeks or less allowed for the return of 80% of normal digital motion, whereas only 66% of normal motion resulted following immobilization for more than 4 weeks. The inability to return to normal motion after phalanx fracture is even greater as the age of the patients increases.[20] Most nondisplaced phalangeal fractures can be treated by neighbor splinting (buddy taping) and early mobilization; displaced transverse mid shaft fractures, spiral fractures, and intra-articular fractures may require open reduction, internal fixation.[7]

METACARPOPHALANGEAL JOINT AND METACARPAL INJURIES
Metacarpophalangeal Joint Dislocations and Ligament Injuries

Second-fifth MCP joints
MCP dislocations are less common than interphalangeal joint dislocations due to the relatively shielded location of these joints from athletic trauma; furthermore, in addition to the stability provided by the volar plate and collateral ligaments, support is also provided from the deep transverse metacarpal ligaments.[21] The index finger is the most commonly affected. Forces that place the finger into hyperextension or ulnar deviation are the usual cause of MCP joint dislocation. Hyperextension injuries rupture the volar plate and result in dorsal subluxation or dislocation. Patients usually present with the affected MCP joint held in extension and the interphalangeal joints held in flexion (**Fig. 11**).[15] Lateral and oblique radiographic views are most important for making the diagnosis of MCP joint dislocation; however, a common pitfall is the overlap of bones

on the lateral view, resulting in MCP dislocations being overlooked. The volar plate or sesamoid bone may become entrapped within the MCP joint following dislocation, which precludes closed reduction of a dislocated MCP joint. Lateral subluxation/dislocation of the MCP joint is less common and typically results from ulnar deviation of the finger with injury to the RCL. Radiographs may reveal an associated avulsion fracture. If no

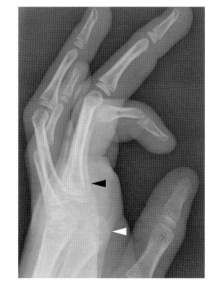

Fig. 11. A 9-year-old boy presents with hand pain and deformity following injury. Lateral radiograph shows dorsal dislocation of the proximal phalanx of the index finger (*black arrowhead*) relative to the head of the second metacarpal (*white arrowhead*). Note the associated flexion of the interphalangeal joints of the index finger.

fracture or malalignment is evident, the only radiographic finding of collateral ligament injury may be adjacent soft tissue swelling. Volar dislocation is rare.

The extensor hood of the finger MCP joint is composed of the extensor digitorum tendon and sagittal bands, which extend from the tendon to the volar plate. Boxer's knuckle, caused by a direct blow to a clenched fist, can result in injury to the extensor hood/sagittal band, with dislocation or subluxation of the central tendon. This dislocation or subluxation results in ulnar subluxation of the MCP joint, which can be seen radiographically on oblique and PA views. The patient presents with pain over their MCP joint from the snapping of the extensor tendon as it subluxes ulnarly with MCP joint flexion as well as loss of motion at the MCP joint. This injury is best treated acutely by buddy taping the affected finger to the neighboring digit or by splinting the hand with the MCP joint held in full extension.[22] Boxer's knuckle represents another example of an injury that if diagnosed at the time of injury can be managed nonoperatively versus requiring surgical fixation if the injury is missed initially (∼3 weeks or more from the time of injury). This diagnosis is frequently misdiagnosed as a trigger finger, because the snapping sensation of the finger is a similar symptom.

Thumb MCP joint

Collateral ligaments serve to stabilize the first MCP joint. The ulnar and RCLs extend from the dorsal aspect of the ulnar and radial condyles on the first metacarpal head to the volar plate and base of the proximal phalanx.[7] In between these 2 collateral ligaments is the dorsal capsule. An accessory collateral ligament attaches to the first metacarpal head volar and proximal to the ulnar collateral ligament (UCL) attachment and inserts distally on the volar plate.[7] The radial and ulnar sesamoid bones are located within the distal aspect of the volar plate.

The UCL is more frequently injured than the RCL because valgus stress injuries are more common than varus stress injuries.[7] UCL injury has traditionally been termed, "gamekeeper's thumb," because it was described originally in Scottish gamekeepers who sustained repetitive minor injury to the ligament by breaking the necks of rabbits, resulting in chronic laxity.[23] In modern times, skiing injuries are a common cause of trauma to the UCL, occurring when the skier falls while holding a ski pole with the affected hand.[9] The injury has also been described in football players, baseball players, hockey players, and wrestlers.[16] The UCL is injured because of forced abduction and radially directed forces at the

MCP joint with hyperextension of the proximal phalanx. Clinically, a patient with an acute gamekeeper's thumb will present with a swollen, painful ulnar aspect of the thumb. Inspection of the hand commonly reveals ecchymosis as well as tenderness to palpation along the ulnar aspect of the MCP joint. On physical examination, the diagnosis is made by testing the UCL. This testing is performed by applying radially and ulnarly directed stresses to the MCP joint. The stress should be applied both with the MCP joint flexed to 30° flexion and with the MCP joint in full extension. Thirty degrees of laxity with the MCP joint in full extension and flexed to 30°, as well as 15° of increased laxity in comparison to the contralateral side, is strongly suggestive of complete injury of the UCL. Lack of a strong end point with ulnarly applied stress can also be used to determine the integrity of the UCL.[24] If laxity is present, but the strong endpoint remains, this is thought to correspond to a partial UCL tear. In additional, the patient's adductor aponeurosis should be palpated. Tenderness in this area suggests the presence of a Stener lesion, in which the thumb adductor aponeurosis becomes entrapped between the avulsed UCL and the base of the proximal phalanx, inhibiting healing of the ligament. Acute treatment of a UCL injury involves placing the patient in a thumb spica splint with the IP joint left free to move and arranging for follow-up with a hand surgeon. Correct diagnosis and treatment of a complete UCL injury in the acute period allow for the option of surgical repair, whereas with the chronically injured MCP joint, UCL reconstruction is often required.[25]

If UCL injury is suspected, AP (or PA), oblique, and lateral radiographs of the thumb are recommended before stress testing to exclude an avulsion fracture that might become displaced with stress. The insertion of the UCL on the proximal phalanx is the most common site of injury; hence, avulsion fractures typically occur at this location, along the ulnar aspect of the base of the proximal phalanx (**Fig. 12**). This bone fragment also marks the site of the retracted UCL. In the absence of an avulsion fracture, radiographs may only reveal slight radial deviation or volar subluxation of the proximal phalanx. If the initial radiographs do not demonstrate any abnormality, stress views (ie, application of stress with the adjacent index finger) of the injured and noninjured thumbs can be obtained,[7] although such views are somewhat controversial. UCL injury is suggested if stress radiographs demonstrate asymmetric widening or subluxation at the MCP joint. UCL injury with accompanying volar subluxation of the proximal phalanx indicates instability that can lead to

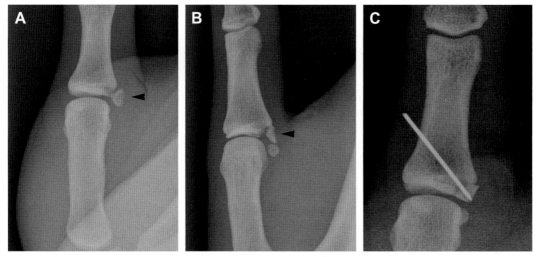

Fig. 12. A 23-year-old man who presents for care following a football injury to his thumb. PA (*A*) and oblique (*B*) radiographs show a bone fragment (*arrowhead*) adjacent to the ulnar aspect of the MCP joint representing an ulnar collateral ligament avulsion fracture fragment arising from the base of the proximal phalanx, with over 90° of clockwise rotation. (*C*) PA radiograph obtained following surgery shows pin fixation of the fracture.

degenerative arthritic changes of the MCP joint if left untreated. Proximal displacement of an avulsion fracture fragment can indicate a Stener lesion on radiographs; however, MRI or ultrasonography may be necessary for diagnosis in the absence of a fracture.

RCL injury at the thumb MCP joint is much less common than UCL injury,[7] although RCL and UCL injuries may occur simultaneously.[6] Acute injuries result from forced and sudden adduction of the MCP joint.[26] Examination should stress the ligament in full extension and 30° of flexion, and suspected injuries should be immobilized in a short-arm thumb spica splint with the IP joint left free to move. Varus stresses to the thumb are much less common than valgus stresses, making the RCL of lesser functional importance.[27] Acute RCL injury can present radiographically with a small avulsion fragment along the radial aspect of the base of the proximal phalanx (**Fig. 13**) with or without volar subluxation of the radial aspect of the MCP joint. However, as these lesions are rare, they often are underdiagnosed and instead present with chronic radiographic findings of degenerative arthritis. An equivalent of a Stener lesion has not been reported with RCL injuries. Surgical repair of the RCL is much less common than UCL injuries; however, these injuries should still be referred to a hand surgeon for close evaluation and follow-up.

Injury to the MCP joint of the thumb resulting in subluxation or dislocation is closely associated with collateral ligament injury. Dorsal dislocations of the thumb MCP joint are more common than volar dislocations (as with finger MCP joint

dislocations) and are most commonly caused by hyperextension injury with rupture of the volar plate.[8]

Metacarpal Fractures

Second-fifth metacarpals

Sports injuries are the most common cause of metacarpal fracture, with the fifth metacarpal being the most commonly fractured.[28] Fourth

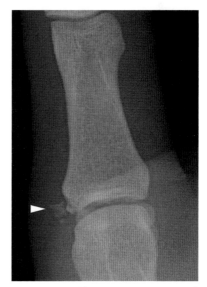

Fig. 13. A 20-year-old man who presents for care following a football injury to his thumb. Radiograph shows small bone fragments adjacent to the radial aspect of the MCP joint, representing a radial collateral ligament avulsion fracture arising from the base of the proximal phalanx. Treatment for small avulsion fractures such as this one is nonoperative.

and fifth metacarpal fractures are more common than second and third metacarpal fractures as there is greater mobility at the fourth and fifth carpometacarpal (CMC) joints than the second and third CMC joints, which in turn makes them more susceptible to trauma and fracture. Rotatory motion at the fifth CMC joint makes the fifth metacarpal even more susceptible to trauma. Deviation forces to the flexed finger can translate to rotational forces to the metacarpal, resulting in spiral fractures. Most metacarpal fractures resulting from athletic trauma, however, are stable.[8]

Metacarpal head fractures are most common at the index finger, followed by the fifth digit.[28] These metacarpal head fractures are associated with low-energy sports trauma (for example, football and basketball).[6] These fractures are generally intra-articular, with comminuted fractures most common and associated with MCP joint subluxation. Horizontal metacarpal head fractures can also occur, which can result in osteonecrosis, especially when displaced.[7] The Brewerton or "ball-catchers" view can be considered for evaluation of metacarpal head fractures when clinical suspicion is high and routine radiographic views do not demonstrate fracture. Alternatively, the hand may be positioned in slight (10–30°) pronation for better evaluation of the second metacarpal, or slight (10–30°) supination for better evaluation of the fourth and fifth metacarpals.[2] Displaced and/or comminuted fractures warrant orthopedic referral.

The most common fifth (and fourth) metacarpal fracture occurs at the metacarpal neck and is termed the "boxer fracture." Although the fracture is most commonly seen in young men who sustained the injury while punching with a clenched fist, it is rarely seen in boxers.[2] This "boxer fracture" is a horizontally oriented, impacted fracture with varying degrees of volar angulation of the distal fracture fragment, and often volar comminution (**Fig. 14**). Greater degrees of angulation are tolerated the more distal the fracture lies. Furthermore, greater angulation (up to 40°–50°) can be tolerated in the fourth and fifth metacarpals because of compensatory flexion/extension motion at the fourth and fifth CMC joints; however, the lack of motion at the second and third CMC joints makes more than 15° of angulation of fractures of the second and third metacarpals unacceptable,[2,6] and in general, such fractures warrant orthopedic referral. Radiologists should keep in mind that the normal metacarpal neck angle is approximately 15°, which can be subtracted from the measured angle to yield the true angular deformity.[2] Rotational malalignment also warrants orthopedic referral. Closed reduction of

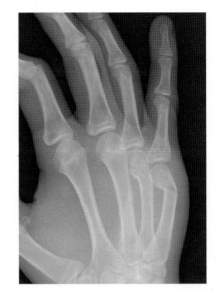

Fig. 14. A 14-year-old boy who presents for care following injury to his hand. Oblique radiograph shows "boxer fractures" of the fourth and fifth metacarpal necks with volar angulation of the distal fracture fragments. Up to 40° to 50° of angulation of the fourth and fifth metacarpals can be tolerated, and hence, this patient was treated nonoperatively with a splint.

a boxer fracture is indicated if the fracture is deformed greater than the accepted angulation. Following reduction, the patient's hand is immobilized in an ulnar gutter splint with the fourth and fifth fingers held in extension at the PIP and DIP joints, flexed to 70° to 80° at the MCP joints, and the wrist in approximately 30° of extension. Typically metacarpal shaft and metacarpal neck fractures will require 3 to 4 weeks of immobilization to allow for healing.

Metacarpal shaft fractures may be transverse, oblique/spiral, or comminuted. Transverse and short-oblique fractures are usually minimally displaced.[16] Minimally displaced mid diaphyseal fractures of the fourth and fifth metacarpals, and nondisplaced fractures of the second and third metacarpals, can be treated with external immobilization[2]; however, metacarpal diaphyseal fractures can be associated with volar angulation of the distal fracture fragment (**Fig. 15**), with MCP joint hyperextension and PIP joint flexion ("claw deformity"),[7] warranting orthopedic referral. Longer oblique and spiral fractures are more prone to rotation and shortening, with up to 5 mm considered to be acceptable; shortening greater than 5 mm, rotation, and angulation may require open reduction and internal fixation (**Fig. 16**).[2,6,16] Comminuted fractures are generally unstable, requiring rigid fixation. The presence of multiple

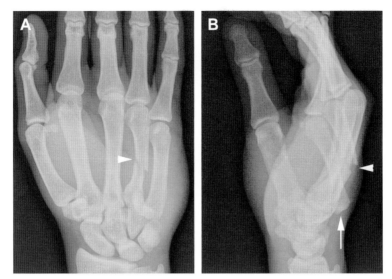

Fig. 15. A 19-year-old man who presents for care following a wrestling injury to his hand. PA (*A*) and lateral (*B*) radiographs of the hand show a transverse fracture of the fourth metacarpal (*arrowhead*) with dorsal apex angulation. Note the associated dorsal dislocation of the base of the fifth metacarpal (*arrow*), best seen on the lateral view. Patients with unstable injuries such as this are referred for operative management.

metacarpal fractures in the same hand is also an indication for surgical fixation.

Isolated fractures of the proximal metacarpal are usually minimally displaced and stable owing to the proximal intermetacarpal ligaments. However, radiographs must be evaluated carefully for intra-articular extension (which can result in osteoarthrosis) as well as disruption of the CMC joint. Fractures of the base of the fifth metacarpal are particularly prone to CMC joint dislocation. Such fractures are the result of an indirect force transmitted from an initial force to the fifth metacarpal head, resulting in a comminuted or bipartite intra-articular fracture at the base of the fifth metacarpal. These fractures are analogous to the Rolando and Bennett fractures of the thumb (see later discussion) (**Fig. 17**). These fractures are unstable, because the pull of the extensor carpi

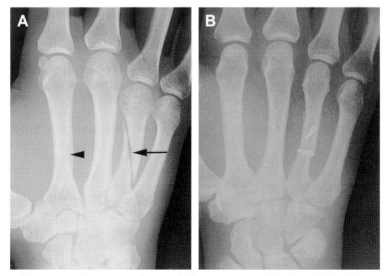

Fig. 16. A 31-year-old woman who presents for care following injury to her hand. (*A*) Oblique radiograph of the hand shows a nondisplaced oblique fracture of the second metacarpal (*arrowhead*) and a displaced long oblique fracture of the fourth metacarpal (*arrow*), resulting in shortening of the bone. The patient underwent open reduction and internal fixation of the unstable fourth metacarpal fracture, restoring the alignment and length of the bone, as shown on the PA radiograph (*B*) obtained following surgery.

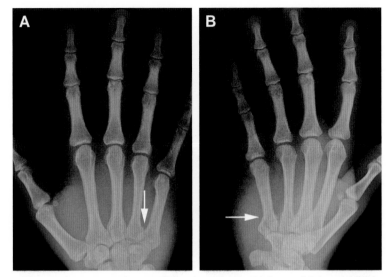

Fig. 17. A 21-year-old man who presents for care following a football injury to his hand. (*A*) PA radiograph of the hand shows a fracture (*arrow*) of the base of the fifth metacarpal that is obscured by the base of the fourth metacarpal. (*B*) Supinated oblique view of the hand better demonstrates the intraarticular fracture (*arrow*).

ulnaris can result in proximal displacement of the fifth metacarpal shaft; pull of the hypothenar muscles can result in radial displacement of the metacarpal shaft as well. Over time, if untreated, this can result in a loss of grip strength and deformity.[7] Despite their seriousness, fifth metacarpal base fractures can be missed on PA radiographs because of the overlying hamate; therefore, careful assessment of the oblique view is required to visualize not only metacarpal base fractures but also associated CMC joint dislocations. Dorsal dislocation of the fifth CMC joint is more common than volar dislocation.[28] The CMC joints should be seen in profile on the frontal view without overlap of apposing articular surfaces.[7] A CMC joint not seen in profile implies that the joint is dislocated. If the fifth CMC joint cannot be visualized fully or there is any question as to whether or not the CMC joint is dislocated, a supinated oblique radiograph or a CT scan of the hand may be considered.

Inspection of rotation and angulation of the digits are key components when evaluating a patient with a metacarpal or phalangeal fracture. When flexing the MCP and PIP joints, each digit should be oriented toward the scaphoid tubercle. Any "scissoring," or crossing over of the fingers, is suggestive of malalignment and possible need for surgical fixation. Alignment of the fingers will often look acceptable with the fingers in full extension, but with the formation of a fist, gross rotation or angulation becomes noticeable. Inspection of the alignment of the fingers of the contralateral hand, if uninjured, provides a good marker of

normal alignment and rotation for each patient. Acutely, these patients should have their fingers splinted with the MCP joints flexed to 80° to 90° and the wrist extended 30° to prevent contracture of the collateral ligaments and subsequent stiffness. This position is known as the "safe position" or intrinsic–plus position and is a useful position for immobilization for most of the injuries of the hand and fingers.[29] It is also very important to inspect the skin and soft tissues carefully around the MCP joint to evaluate for the possibility of an open fracture or "fight bite" depending on the mechanism of injury.[11]

First metacarpal

Thumb metacarpal fractures can result in severe disability (osteoarthritis and malunion) if left untreated. Thumb metacarpal fractures represent 20% of all metacarpal fractures, with most occurring at the metacarpal base[28] as a result of an axial load directed against the flexed metacarpal (for example, when a quarterback's throwing hand strikes an opponent's helmet during follow-through).[12] Three main types of thumb metacarpal base fractures have been characterized: intra-articular 2-part, intra-articular comminuted, and extraarticular.

A 2-part intra-articular fracture of the base of the first metacarpal is also known as a Bennett fracture and represents the most common fracture of the first metacarpal (**Fig. 18**). The injury usually consists of an oblique or vertical fracture plane extending through the volar aspect of the base of the thumb from the metaphyseal-diaphyseal junction

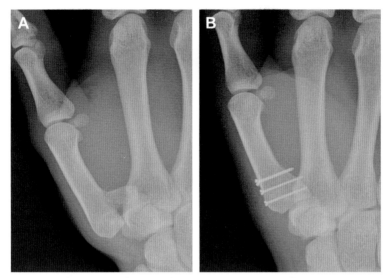

Fig. 18. A 26-year-old man who presents for care after sustaining a Bennett fracture-dislocation while biking. (*A*) PA radiograph shows an intra-articular fracture of the base of the first metacarpal with angulation of the volar-ulnar fragment and dorsoradial dislocation of the remainder of the metacarpal. (*B*) Postoperative radiograph shows reduction and fixation of the fracture-dislocation.

to the joint surface and is associated with disruption of the stabilizing ligaments of the CMC joint. This injury results in a volar/ulnar fracture fragment that remains attached to the trapezium via the volar beak ligament, whereas the remainder of the metacarpal is dislocated dorsally and radially by the abductor pollicis longus. Dislocation of the first CMC joint without fracture is rare and involves rupture of the volar beak ligament with dorsal displacement of the first metacarpal.[8] If gross instability exists or reduction cannot be achieved, open reduction and reconstruction of the volar ligament are performed; this procedure may be undertaken in chronic cases or acutely in the high-performance athlete (eg, a quarterback's throwing hand).[8]

Comminuted intra-articular fractures through the base of the thumb are termed "Rolando fractures" (**Fig. 19**) and are less common than Bennett fractures. These fractures may have a Y or T configuration, or be more severely comminuted; up to 50% of these fractures result in osteoarthritis.[7] As with Bennett fractures, Rolando fractures disrupt the CMC joint, stabilizing ligaments, and dislocation or subluxation of the CMC joint is a common associated finding, although proximal displacement of the larger metacarpal fragment by the abductor pollicis longus may not be as pronounced as with Bennett fractures.

Extra-articular fractures through the base of the thumb can be oblique or transverse in orientation. Oblique fractures can result in additional displacement of the distal metacarpal shaft fracture

fragment because of the pull of the abductor pollicus longus[7] and may require pin fixation. Pin fixation is not typically an issue with transversely oriented fractures; although transverse fractures are often associated with some apex radial angulation, they can generally be managed with closed reduction.

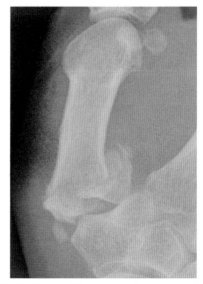

Fig. 19. A 54-year-old woman who presents for care after sustaining an injury to her hand. Thumb radiograph shows a comminuted fracture of the base of the first metacarpal (Rolando fracture), which was treated with closed reduction and percutaneous pinning.

On initial presentation, Bennett fractures, Rolondo fractures, and first metacarpal shaft fractures all receive treatment by immobilization of the affected thumb with a short-arm thumb spica splint. Metacarpal shaft fractures with acceptable fracture alignment can be managed with 4 weeks of immobilization to allow for healing. Because of the great amount of mobility in the thumb, up to 30° of angulation is acceptable for a first metacarpal shaft fracture. Angulation greater than 30° warrants surgical evaluation. Bennett and Rolondo fractures will nearly always require surgical fixation. Severely angled metacarpal shaft fractures, Bennett fractures, and Rolondo fractures can be surgically stabilized with closed reduction and percutaneous pinning versus open reduction and internal fixation with mini-fragment screws.[30]

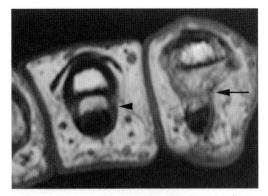

Fig. 20. A 52-year-old man who developed a flexion contracture of his index finger following PIP joint dislocation. T1-weighted transverse MR image of the middle and index fingers through the proximal phalanges shows disruption of the A2 pulley of the index finger (*arrow*). Note the intact A2 pulley (*arrowhead*) of the middle finger stabilizing the flexor tendon apparatus.

Advanced Imaging Considerations

When there is strong clinical concern for fracture following normal or equivocal radiographs, CT can be considered.[3] CT may also be useful for evaluating articular surfaces in the setting of intra-articular fractures, and for confirming or excluding malalignment at the carpometacarpal joints. 2D-reformatted and 3D-reformatted images can aid in preoperative planning for complex intra-articular fractures. Malunion, delayed union, and nonunion of fractures can be assessed with CT. CT also provides the radiologist with information regarding soft tissues of the hand (eg, lacerations, foreign bodies, hematomas, etc), although tendon and ligament injuries are usually better assessed with sonography or MRI. In the setting of athletic trauma, intravenous contrast is generally not indicated.

Although MRI can be used to assess bone marrow, it typically does not provide additional information regarding hand fractures beyond radiographs. MRI can have a role, however, in the evaluation of soft tissue structures. Muscle and tendon injuries, including strains, hematomas, and ruptures, are readily visualized with MRI. Injuries to the pulley mechanism (which stabilizes the flexor tendon apparatus) can be depicted with MRI (**Fig. 20**). MRI has also proven useful for the evaluation of ligaments, including injuries to the UCL of the thumb and associated Stener lesions, as well as volar plate injuries. Ultrasonography can be a reliable alternative to MRI for the depiction of musculotendinous, ligamentous, and pulley injuries. Sonography also benefits from its ability to evaluate tendons dynamically with ease. The ultrasound probe should be held perpendicular to the tendon in question to reduce anisotropy, which can mimic pathologic abnormality.

SUMMARY

Conventional radiographs are the most common modality used to diagnose athletic injuries to the hand. Athletic injuries to the hand can be due to a variety of mechanisms and a variety of sports. The radiologist should be aware of the clinical presentation and radiographic appearance of the injuries discussed in this article to ensure prompt and accurate diagnosis.

REFERENCES

1. De Jonge JJ, Kingma J, van der Lei B, et al. Phalangeal fractures of the hand. An analysis of gender and age-related incidence and aetiology. J Hand Surg Br 1994;19(2):168–70.
2. Capo JT, Hastings H. Metacarpal and phalangeal fractures in athletes. Clin Sports Med 1998;17(3): 491.
3. American College of Radiology. ACR appropriateness criteria®: acute hand and wrist trauma. Available at: http://www.acr.org/SecondaryMainMenuCategories/ quality_safety/app_criteria/pdf/ExpertPanelonMuscul oskeletalImaging/AcuteHandandWristTraumaDoc1. aspx. Accessed April 2, 2012.
4. Wang QC, Johnson BA. Fingertip injuries. Am Fam Physician 2001;63:1961–6.
5. Barton NJ. Fractures of the hand. J Bone Joint Surg Br 1984;66(2):159–67.
6. Rosner JL, Zlatkin MB, Clifford P, et al. Imaging of athletic wrist and hand injuries. Semin Musculoskelet Radiol 2004;8(1):57–79.

7. Jarvik JG, Dalinka MK, Kneeland JB. Hand injuries in adults. Semin Roentgenol 1991;26(4):282–99.

8. Rettig AC. Athletic injuries of the wrist and hand. Am J Sports Med 2004;32(1):262–73.

9. Johnson CA, Yoong E, Chojnowski A, et al. Four hand injuries not to miss: avoiding pitfalls in the emergency department. Eur J Emerg Med 2011; 18:186–91.

10. Leddy JP, Packer JW. Avulsion of the profundus tendon insertion in athletes. J Hand Surg 1977; 2(1):66–9.

11. Green DP, Hotchkiss RN, Pederson WC, et al, editors. Green's operative hand surgery. 5th edition. Philadelphia: Churchill-Livingstone; 2005. p. 281.

12. Rettig ME, Dassa G, Raskin KB. Volar plate arthroplasty of the distal interphalangeal joint. J Hand Surg 2001;26(5):940–4.

13. Itadera E, Muramatsu Y, Hiwatari R, et al. Chronic recurrent dislocation of the distal interphalangeal joint of the finger: case report. J Hand Surg Am 2009;34:1091–3.

14. Banerji S, Bullocks J, Cole P, et al. Irreducible distal interphalangeal joint dislocation. Ann Plast Surg 2007;58(6):683–5.

15. Calfee RP, Sommerkamp TG. Fracture-dislocation about the finger joints. J Hand Surg 2009;34:1140–7.

16. McCue FC, Baugher WH, Kulund DN, et al. Hand and wrist injuries in the athlete. Am J Sports Med 1979;7(5):275–86.

17. Bekler H, Gokce A, Beyzadeoglu T. Avulsion fractures from the base of the phalanges of the fingers. Tech Hand Up Extrem Surg 2006;10(3):157–61.

18. Leggit JC, Meko CJ. Acute finger injuries: part II. Fractures, dislocations, and thumb injuries. Am Fam Physician 2006;73(5):827–34.

19. Kiefhaber TR, Stern PJ. Fracture dislocations of the proximal interphalangeal joint. J Hand Surg 1998; 23(3):368–80.

20. Strickland JW. Phalangeal fractures: factors influencing digit performance. Orthop Rev 1982;11:39–50.

21. Fultz CW, Buchanan JR. Complex fracture-dislocation of the metacarpophalangeal joint. Clin Orthop Relat Res 1988;227:255–60.

22. Araki S, Ohtani T, Tanaka T. Acute dislocations of the extensor digitorum communis tendon at the metacarpalphalangeal joint. a report of five cases. J Bone Joint Surg Am 1987;69(4):616–9.

23. Campbell CS. Gamekeeper's thumb. J Bone Joint Surg Br 1955;37:148–9.

24. Tang P. Collateral ligament injuries of the thumb metacarpophalangeal joint. J Am Acad Orthop Surg 2011;19(5):287–96.

25. Arnold DM, Cooney WP, Wood MB. Surgical management of chronic ulnar collateral ligament insufficiency of the thumb metacarpophalangeal joint. Orthop Rev 1992;21(5):583–8.

26. Posner MA, Retaillaud JL. Metacarpophalangeal joint injuries of the thumb. Hand Clin 1992;8:713–32.

27. Edelstein DM, Kardashian G, Lee SK. Radial collateral ligament injuries of the thumb. J Hand Surg Am 2008;33:760–70.

28. Stanton JS, Dias JJ, Burke FD. Fractures of the tubular bones of the hand. J Hand Surg Eur Vol 2007;32:626–36.

29. Kozin SH, Thoder JJ, Lieberman G. Operative treatment of metacarpal and phalangeal shaft fractures. J Am Acad Orthop Surg 2000;8(2):111–21.

30. Soyer AD. Fractures of the base of the first metacarpal: current treatment options. J Am Acad Orthop Surg 1999;7:403–12.

Throwing Injuries of the Upper Extremity

Neel B. Patel, MD[a],*, Stephen Thomas, MD[a],
Martin L. Lazarus, MD[b,c]

KEYWORDS

- Shoulder • Elbow • Throwing • Sports • MR imaging • MR arthrography

KEY POINTS

- Knowledge of the kinetics and kinematics of the pitching motion is integral in understanding shoulder and elbow injuries in the overhead thrower.
- The majority of injuries in the overhead thrower occur during the late cocking, acceleration, and deceleration phases of the pitching motion.
- Magnetic resonance arthrography increases sensitivity for detecting ligamentous, tendinous, and labral abnormality in the overhead thrower.
- Imaging findings must be correlated with the overhead thrower's symptoms, as some imaging abnormalities may not be the source of clinical symptoms.

INTRODUCTION

Overhead throwing imparts high-tensile loads to an athlete's upper extremity, risking injury to the shoulder or elbow. Although overhead throwing in baseball serves as the prototypical model, similar injuries occur in softball, tennis, football, and track and field, particularly in javelin throwers. Repetitive throwing subjects the shoulder and elbow to extreme positions with excessive multidirectional stresses, with a wide spectrum of abnormalities affecting both joints. This article reviews the overhead throwing motion and the injuries that can occur during each particular phase of throwing.

PITCHING MOTION

The "kinetic chain" describes a sequence of coordinated events that occurs during the overhead pitching motion.[1] Kinetic energy is transferred from the lower extremity and trunk to the upper extremity, allowing the pitcher to propel a baseball with velocities approaching 100 miles per hour.

The overhead pitching motion takes less than 2 seconds and is divided into 6 phases: wind-up, early cocking, late cocking, acceleration, deceleration, and follow-through.[2–5] The majority of shoulder and elbow injuries occur during the late cocking, acceleration, and deceleration phases.

Phase I: Wind-Up

The wind-up is highly variable among pitchers; it begins when the pitcher initiates motion and ends when the ball is removed from the glove. The wind-up primarily prepares the pitcher for the subsequent phases of throwing, and there is a large variation in movement to accommodate individual throwing styles. At the end of this phase, the shoulder and elbow experience minimal muscle activity and forces.[4,6]

Phase II: Early Cocking (Stride)

In the early cocking phase, the pitcher extends the stride leg toward the batter and lowers the center of

Disclosures: None.
[a] Department of Radiology, University of Chicago Medical Center, 5841 South Maryland Avenue, MC2026, Chicago, IL 60637, USA; [b] Department of Radiology, Evanston Hospital, NorthShore University Healthsystem, 2650 Ridge Avenue, Evanston, IL 60201, USA; [c] The University of Chicago, Pritzker School of Medicine, 924 East 57th Street, Suite 104, Chicago, IL 60637-5415, USA
* Corresponding author.
E-mail address: Neel.Patel2@uchospitals.edu

Radiol Clin N Am 51 (2013) 257–277
http://dx.doi.org/10.1016/j.rcl.2012.09.016

gravity. The trunk is kept as far posterior as possible to maximize the potential for rotation and contribution to pitch velocity.[2] The throwing shoulder is in approximately 90° of abduction, 15° to 30° of horizontal abduction, and 50° of external rotation, while the elbow reaches approximately 85° of flexion.[3–5] The inferior glenohumeral ligament limits anterior and posterior translation of the humeral head relative to the glenoid during 90° of abduction.[7] The trapezius, serratus anterior, deltoid, supraspinatus, infraspinatus, and teres minor muscles are all activated during this phase.[3,5]

Phase III: Late Cocking

Late cocking begins after the stride foot is planted and ends with the shoulder in maximum shoulder external rotation of 160° to 180°.[8,9] Shoulder abduction of 90° (from the early cocking phase) combined with maximum external rotation in the late cocking phase results in posterior translation of the humeral head on the glenoid.[10] Rotation of the torso generates 650 N of rotator cuff compressive force and 400 N of shear force across the anterior shoulder.[3] The long head of the biceps limits anterior translation of the humeral head. Internal impingement and injuries to the rotator cuff, biceps, and type II superior labrum anterior-posterior (SLAP) tears may all occur during this phase.

To prevent valgus extension and excessive external rotation, the elbow generates a varus force of between 64 and 120 N·m through the combined actions of the ulnar collateral ligament (UCL), wrist flexor-pronator group, anconeus, and triceps.[4] The UCL is theoretically overloaded as it receives an estimated force of 35 N·m, which is beyond its maximal load bearing capacity of 32 N·m measured in cadaveric studies.[11] Elbow injuries primarily occur during the late cocking and acceleration phase because of eventual failure to counteract large valgus forces across the joint.

Phase IV: Acceleration

Acceleration internally rotates the shoulder from maximal external rotation of 160° to 180° to the point of ball release at 90° to 100° of external rotation.[5,12] This internal rotation is one of the fastest human motions, with mean maximum angular velocity approaching 7000°/s and internal rotary torque of approximately 15,000 in-lb (1695 N·m).[2,13] Activation of the latissimus dorsi and pectoralis major are the primary contributors to pitching velocity.[6] During horizontal adduction to the neutral position, 50 N of shear stress across the posterior shoulder helps recenter the humeral head.[5,6]

Centrifugal force during acceleration attempts to distract the forearm from the elbow, but a compressive force of 500 to 780 N at the lateral radiocapitellar joint maintains elbow integrity throughout the late cocking and acceleration phase.[4,12] The wrist flexor-pronator group is very active at ball release as the pitcher applies spin on the ball.[14] Most injuries to the elbow occur in this phase along with the late cocking phase.

Phase V: Deceleration

Deceleration is the most violent phase of pitching and is a reversal of the first 3 phases of the pitching motion. Deceleration begins with ball release and ends when the shoulder is at maximum internal rotation and adducted across the chest.[14] The musculature of the shoulder girdle and the rotator cuff eccentrically contract to slow down shoulder rotation with posterior shear forces of 400 N, inferior shear forces of 300 N, and compressive forces greater than 1000 N.[3] These strong forces may lead to type II SLAP lesions, Bennett lesions, posterior instability, and rotator cuff tears due to impingement.

Phase VI: Follow-Through

The follow-through begins when the shoulder is at maximum internal rotation, and is an important phase in which injuries can be minimized. Muscle activity and joint loads decrease; however, compressive and shear forces remain across the shoulder.[12] A longer follow-through will dissipate more stress through the trunk and lower extremity, decreasing the peak load to the posterior rotator cuff and reducing risk of injury.[14]

IMAGING OF THE SHOULDER

Magnetic resonance (MR) imaging is the preferred modality for evaluating the shoulder because of its multiplanar imaging capability, excellent soft-tissue contrast, and lack of radiation exposure. Imaging may be performed with a variety of MR units, ranging from low-field open 0.2-T to high-field closed 3.0-T systems. High–field-strength systems provide a higher signal-to-noise ratio (SNR), allowing faster imaging, decreased motion artifact, thinner slice thickness, and better spatial resolution than low-field-strength systems. Low–field-strength systems produce less imaging artifacts and allow imaging of claustrophobic patients. Most studies comparing the 2 systems have shown similar diagnostic accuracy in evaluating the shoulder, whereas others have found superior performance characteristics with high–field-strength systems.[15–18]

The patient is positioned supine with the arm at the side, ideally in external rotation for optimal visualization of the rotator-cuff tendons, biceps-labral complex, and inferior glenohumeral ligament.[19,20] A dedicated surface coil is placed on the shoulder to optimize SNR. Specific imaging protocols vary by imaging system (field strength, coil capability) and institution, but generally include coronal oblique, sagittal oblique, and axial images.

Axial images are obtained from above the acromion to below the glenohumeral joint. Coronal oblique images are oriented parallel to the supraspinatus tendon as seen on the axial images, and the sagittal oblique images are oriented perpendicular to the coronal images. The standard unenhanced MR imaging protocol includes axial spoiled gradient-echo, fat-saturated axial proton-density (PD), coronal oblique PD, fat-saturated coronal oblique T2-weighted (T2W), sagittal oblique T1-weighted (T1W), and fat-saturated sagittal oblique T2W sequences.

Direct MR arthrography with injection of gadolinium contrast (gadodiamide) (Omniscan; GE Healthcare, Waukesha, WI) into the glenohumeral joint allows distension of the joint capsule with optimal visualization of the intra-articular structures. The solution contains a 50:50 mixture of dilute gadolinium (0.4 mL in a 50-mL bag of saline) and iodinated contrast material (Omnipaque 240; GE Healthcare). The patient is placed supine with the arm in external rotation, and the medial cortex of the humeral head is targeted via an anterior approach under fluoroscopic guidance. The skin and soft tissues are anesthetized with 1% lidocaine. Approximately 12 mL of dilute gadolinium/iodinated contrast mixture is injected into the glenohumeral joint with a 22-gauge spinal needle.

The standard direct MR arthrography protocol includes fat-saturated axial T1W, fat-saturated coronal oblique T1W, fat-saturated coronal oblique T2W, coronal oblique PD, and fat-saturated sagittal oblique PD sequences. The sensitivity of detecting partial-thickness rotator-cuff tears and labral tears are increased when imaging is performed with the patient's arm in abduction and external rotation (ABER).[21–23] The ABER position reduces tension on the rotator cuff, allowing intra-articular contrast to flow more easily into a tear, increasing sensitivity for detection.[24] In the throwing athlete, the ABER view simulates the position of the shoulder in the late cocking phase of throwing and can help diagnose SLAP tears.

ROTATOR-CUFF INJURIES

Rotator-cuff injury can occur during multiple phases of the overhead throwing motion. Injury may occur during the late cocking phase because of anterior instability, during the acceleration phase because of subacromial impingement, and from the cumulative effects of repetitive microtrauma from throwing.[25] MR arthrography is more sensitive and more specific than unenhanced MR imaging or ultrasonography for the detection of rotator-cuff injury.[26] Partial-thickness rotator-cuff tears are more common than full-thickness tears, and usually occur as articular-sided tears at the junction of the supraspinatus and infraspinatus tendons. The rotator cuff works together with the labrum and the glenohumeral ligaments to restrain excessive motion, and combined injuries are also possible.

Partial-thickness rotator-cuff tears can be classified by their position as either articular, bursal, or intrasubstance, and are further graded by thickness of involvement, assuming a normal rotator-cuff thickness of 10 to 12 mm: grade I (<3 mm), grade II (3–6 mm), and grade III (>6 mm).[27,28]

Overuse Injuries

Overuse injury to the rotator cuff usually occurs in the absence of impingement. The rotator cuff resists horizontal adduction, internal rotation, and distraction forces during the deceleration phase of throwing.[3] Repetitive stress may speed up normal degeneration and lead to rotator-cuff failure and injury.[29]

Partial articular-sided tendon avulsion (PASTA) and rim-rent rotator-cuff tears describe partial-thickness articular surface tears adjacent to the insertion on the greater tuberosity that may involve fibers of the supraspinatus and/or infraspinatus tendons.[30–32] This region is vulnerable to tearing, as it is inherently weak because collagen fibers make an abrupt 90° turn toward the greater tuberosity.[33] These tears are best seen on T2W images with fluid-intensity signal involving the tendon without a gap (**Fig. 1**). Supraspinatus rim-rent tears may involve the anteriormost fibers of the rotator cuff and may be missed if the shoulder is imaged in marked internal rotation, as the anterior cuff is difficult to visualize on sagittal oblique sequences (**Fig. 1**).[30] These lesions may progress to full-thickness tears if they are not recognized early. Partial articular tears with intratendinous extension (PAINT) lesions, increasingly seen in overhead-throwing athletes, occur at the junction of the posterior supraspinatus and the superior infraspinatus tendons with longitudinal propagation into the substance of the tendon (**Fig. 2**).[34]

Subacromial Impingement

Subacromial impingement may be divided into two categories: primary and secondary. Primary

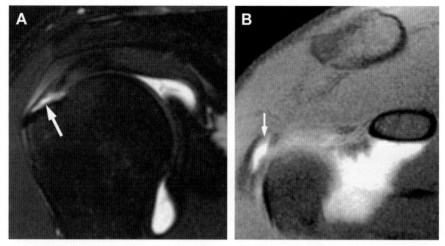

Fig. 1. Rim-rent/PASTA (partial articular-sided tendon avulsion) lesions. (*A*) Fat-saturated T2-weighted (T2W) coronal oblique MR image with intra-articular gadolinium shows high signal (*arrow*) extending between the greater tuberosity and the distal articular surface of the supraspinatus tendon. (*B*) Fat-saturated T1-weighted (T1W) coronal oblique MR image with intra-articular gadolinium in another patient shows gadolinium signal (*arrow*) in the far anterior fibers of the supraspinatus tendon, indicating a partial-thickness tear.

subcromial impingement describes extrinsic compression of the subacromial space, which contains the supraspinatus tendon, tendon of the long head of the biceps, and subacromial bursa. This form of impingement is not common in young athletes, but may occasionally affect throwing athletes older than 35 years.[35] Repetitive overhead

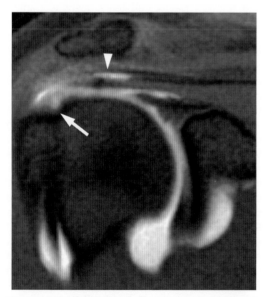

Fig. 2. PAINT (partial articular tears with intratendinous extension) lesion. Fat-saturated T1W coronal oblique MR image with intra-articular gadolinium shows a near full-thickness tear of the supraspinatus tendon near its insertion (*arrow*). Gadolinium extends proximally into the substance of the tendon (*arrowhead*) in longitudinal fashion.

throwing usually leads to osteophyte formation along the inferior surface of the acromion, with subsequent narrowing of the subacromial space. Less common causes of subacromial impingement include variant acromial morphology, persistent os acromiale (**Fig. 3**), or thickening of the coracoacromial ligament. Acromial shape has been classified as flat or type 1, curved or type 2, and hooked or type 3, with type 3 acromion associated with rotator-cuff tears.[36] A persistent os acromiale should not be diagnosed before 25 years of age, as a normal physis can persist until this age.[37]

Secondary subacromial impingement is due to inherent instability of the humeral head within the glenoid, and is one of the most common forms of impingement in overhead-throwing athletes.[38] The anatomic abnormalities associated with primary subacrominal impingement are not present. Rather, repetitive microtrauma from maximal external rotation and horizontal adduction during the late cocking phase can result in ligamentous laxity, leading to anterior instability.[5] With prolonged anterior instability, the rotator-cuff muscles become fatigued and can no longer prevent further anterior translation of the humeral head, leading to rotator-cuff tears.

Rotator-cuff injuries with primary impingement usually occur in the anterior portion of the supraspinatus, however with secondary impingement, injuries can occur anywhere in the supraspinatus or infraspinatus tendons.[33] Differentiating between the two types of subacrominal impingement is imperative, as primary impingement is treated with coracoacrominal decompression and secondary

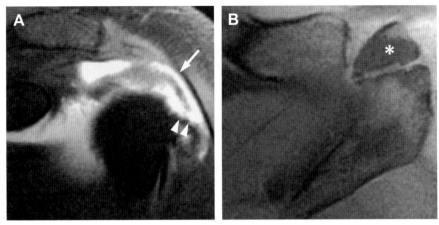

Fig. 3. Primary subacromial impingement. (*A*) Fat-saturated T1W coronal oblique MR image with intra-articular gadolinium shows a full-thickness tear (*arrowheads*) of the anterior supraspinatus tendon at its attachment to the greater tuberosity with minimal tendinous retraction. Gadolinium contrast traverses the tear and fills the subdeltoid/subacromial bursa (*arrow*). (*B*) Fat-saturated T1W axial MR image shows an os acromiale (*asterisk*).

impingement is treated with capsuloligamentous laxity correction and labral repair.[39]

Posterosuperior Impingement

During maximal external rotation in the late cocking phase, large stresses are placed on the static and dynamic stabilizers of the anterior shoulder. There is repetitive contact and compression of the posterior supraspinatus and anterior infraspinatus tendons between the humeral head and posterior glenoid.[40] Although this compression is physiologically normal, symptomatic compression can lead to posterosuperior, or internal, impingement.[40]

The mechanism leading to posterosuperior impingement is under debate. Anterior laxity and instability with anterior subluxation of the humeral head may be a contributing factor.[41] Alternatively, the posterior capsular theory suggests that repeated overhead throwing leads to hypertrophy of the infraspinatus and posterior band of the inferior glenohumeral ligament, allowing external hyperrotation of the humeral head and more pronounced internal impingement.[42,43] The subsequent posterior capsular contracture leads to a glenohumeral internal rotation deficit (GIRD). Regardless of the mechanism, the injury pattern of posterosuperior impingement is predictable, and consists of rotator-cuff tears and posterosuperior labral tears.

Posterosuperior impingement may lead to "kissing" lesions, on the glenoid side involving the posterosuperior labrum and subchondral bone and on the humeral side involving the supraspinatus, infraspinatus, and greater tuberosity.[44] MR arthrography is superior to conventional MR imaging for the detection of partial rotator-cuff tears, labral tears, and glenohumeral ligament abnormalities.[45–47] Posterosuperior impingement tears are usually small, partial-thickness articular surfaces that are best seen with ABER positioning with MR arthrography.[45] Additional findings include high–signal-intensity cystic changes on T2W images in the posterosuperior humeral head at the attachment of the infraspinatus and posterior supraspinatus tendons (**Fig. 4**).[48]

Subcoracoid Impingement

Subcoracoid impingement is an uncommon cause of anterior shoulder pain in the throwing athlete that may occur during the deceleration phase of pitching.[44,49] Symptomatic impingement of the subscapularis tendon between the lesser tuberosity of the humeral head and the coracoid process causes dull anteromedial shoulder pain exacerbated by forward elevation, internal rotation, and cross-arm adduction.[50] Initial treatment includes activity modification, avoidance of provocative maneuvers, and physical therapy; however, if conservative treatment fails, surgical decompression with open coracoplasty or coracoid osteotomy may be considered.[50,51]

Subcoracoid impingement is primarily a clinical diagnosis that may be supported or suggested by MR imaging.[52] Giaroli and colleagues[52] found that although a coracohumeral interval of 11.5 mm was statistically significantly related to subcoracoid impingement, it was poorly predictive of the diagnosis. Thus, measurement of the coracohumeral interval is not solely diagnostic. Imaging findings supporting a clinical diagnosis of impingement may include partial-thickness or full-thickness subscapularis tendon tears, or cysts

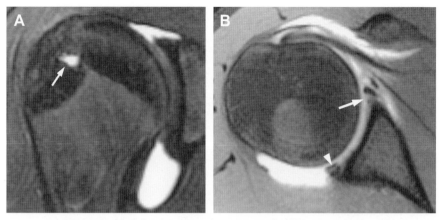

Fig. 4. Posterosuperior impingement. (*A*) Fat-saturated T2W coronal oblique MR image with intra-articular gadolinium shows high-signal cysts (*arrow*) in the posterolateral humeral head. (*B*) Fat-saturated T1W axial MR image with intra-articular gadolinium shows high signal within the anteroinferior labrum (*arrow*) and the posterior labrum (*arrowhead*), compatible with labral tears.

and bone marrow edema in the lesser tuberosity (**Fig. 5**).[53]

LABRUM

The labrum is a fibrocartilaginous rim surrounding the glenoid that functionally deepens the glenoid socket and increases the surface area available for contact with the humeral head. The labrum improves glenohumeral joint stability by centering the humeral head on the glenoid and by maintaining negative intra-articular pressure within the shoulder.[54,55]

Andrews and colleagues[56] first described tears of the anterosuperior labrum near the origin of the long head of the biceps tendon (LHBT) in baseball players. SLAP (superior labrum anterior to posterior) lesions were first classified by Snyder and colleagues[57] into 4 types. Since the original classification, 10 types of SLAP lesions have been described by different investigators.[58–60]

The SLAP type II lesion is a common cause of shoulder pain in the overhead-throwing athlete.[61,62] The lesion consists of stripping of the superior labrum and biceps attachment from the glenoid. The SLAP type II lesion can be further divided into 3 subtypes based on direction of the labral tear: type IIA with anterior extension, type IIB with posterior extension, and type IIC with anterior and posterior extension.[59] SLAP type IIB and IIC lesions can be disabling to overhead throwers because of glenohumeral instability.[63]

Multiple potential mechanisms for this lesion have been described in the literature. A cadaveric

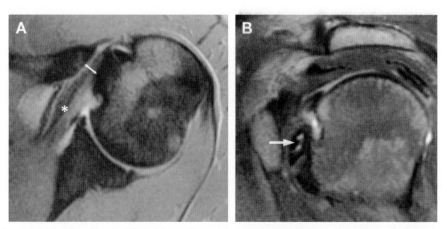

Fig. 5. Subcoracoid impingement. (*A*) Axial gradient-echo MR image shows narrowing of the coracohumeral space (*double-headed arrow*) to less than 6 mm and intermediate signal of thickened subscapularis tendon (*asterisk*). (*B*) Fat-saturated T2W coronal oblique MR image shows high signal (*arrow*), suggestive of interstitial tear, in the central subscapularis tendon.

study has shown that SLAP type II lesions are most likely to occur during the late cocking phase of overhead throwing.[64] Excessive stress on the LHBT during the deceleration phase of throwing led to SLAP type II lesions in a laboratory study using mesh models of the glenoid and labrum.[65] In addition, these lesions are thought to be caused by a peel-back phenomenon whereby twisting of the biceps tendon insertion during shoulder abduction and external rotation causes separation of the posterosuperior labrum from the glenoid.[66] Clinical symptoms include pain, decreased throwing velocity, or intermittent clicking during the cocking phase of throwing.[61,67]

MR imaging is the primary modality for the evaluation of the labrum (**Fig. 6**). SLAP type II lesions are best seen on coronal oblique images as high signal (fluid or intra-articular gadolinium) oriented laterally in the labrum.[63,68] Additional findings include a concurrent anterosuperior labral tear and anteroposterior extension of high signal in the superior labrum on fat-saturated T1W axial images.[63] Sensitivity is increased with imaging in the ABER position on MR arthrography.[23] The normal variant superior sublabral sulcus is a significant cause of a false-positive diagnosis of a SLAP lesion due to overlapping findings on MR imaging, and care must be taken to differentiate the two when evaluating for labral tears.

BICEPS TENDON

The biceps is a common cause of shoulder pain in the overhead-throwing athlete, and is typically injured from overuse. The long head of the biceps contributes to anterior shoulder stability by limiting anterior translation of the humeral head and diminishing stress placed on the inferior glenohumeral ligament during the late cocking phase of throwing.[69] Repetitive overriding of the tendon of the long head of the biceps over the lesser tuberosity can lead to biceps tendonitis.[5,70]

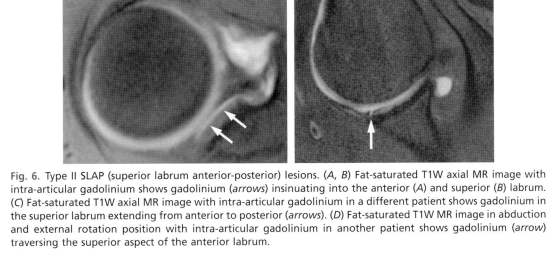

Fig. 6. Type II SLAP (superior labrum anterior-posterior) lesions. (*A, B*) Fat-saturated T1W axial MR image with intra-articular gadolinium shows gadolinium (*arrows*) insinuating into the anterior (*A*) and superior (*B*) labrum. (*C*) Fat-saturated T1W axial MR image with intra-articular gadolinium in a different patient shows gadolinium in the superior labrum extending from anterior to posterior (*arrows*). (*D*) Fat-saturated T1W MR image in abduction and external rotation position with intra-articular gadolinium in another patient shows gadolinium (*arrow*) traversing the superior aspect of the anterior labrum.

The natural history of biceps abnormality probably represents a progressive continuum from tenosynovitis, tendinosis, delamination, and partial tearing, to full-thickness tear.[71] Clinical symptoms of LHBT injury are typically located anteriorly in the shoulder, with pain reproducible by palpation over the bicipital groove.

Located within the rotator interval, the LHBT is located far anteriorly in the shoulder, attaches at the anterior superior labrum, and travels inferiorly in the bicipital groove. The superficial fibers of subscapularis tendon cross the bicipital groove to attach on the greater tuberosity, whereas the deeper fibers of the subscapularis tendon insert on the lesser tuberosity.

MR imaging is the most popular imaging modality for evaluating the LHBT. The sagittal oblique and axial planes provide optimal visualization of the intra-articular LHBT in the rotator interval and the bicipital groove, respectively.[72] Fluid may be present within the dependent aspect of the tendon sheath, which is normal as the tendon sheath communicates with the synovium of the glenohumeral joint. Fluid within the tendon sheath of the long head of the biceps is abnormal if it completely surrounds the tendon in the absence of a joint effusion (**Fig. 7**).[73]

Findings of tendinosis of the LHBT are similar to that of other tendons in the shoulder. Tendinosis and partial-thickness tears are not usually distinguishable on T1W images, as both show intermediate to high signal intensity in a thickened tendon. However on T2W images, intrasubstance signal not as high as fluid signal suggests tendinosis, whereas intrasubstance signal similar to fluid or gadolinium on MR arthrography are characteristic of partial-thickness tears (see **Fig. 7**).[74] Subluxation or dislocation of the LHBT occurs with tears of the subscapularis tear. These lesions are best shown on axial images with an empty bicipital groove and medial displacement of the LHBT into the joint.[75]

BENNETT LESION

Often seen in overhead-throwing athletes, the Bennett lesion is an extra-articular crescent-shaped ossification of the posterior inferior glenoid at the insertion of the posterior band of the inferior glenohumeral ligament.[76,77] The lesion is thought to be found exclusively in baseball players and may be seen in up to 22% of Major League pitchers.[77] The lesion is often associated with posterior labral tears and undersurface rotator-cuff tears.[76,78] Although the mechanism of injury is debated, the Bennett lesion is thought to represent reactive bone formation from repetitive traction on the posterior band of the inferior glenohumeral ligament during the deceleration phase of throwing.[76,79] Some investigators suggest that a posterior labrocapsular periosteal sleeve avulsion (POLPSA) lesion may represent an acute form of a Bennett lesion.[80]

Athletes may present with pain during the cocking and follow-through phases of throwing and may have palpable tenderness along the posterior glenoid.[76] Bennett lesions may be treated with surgical excision; however, no specific criteria exist for routine excision, as solitary Bennett lesions may be asymptomatic and concomitant symptoms of internal impingement are often present.[77]

Bennett lesions may be seen on radiography and computed tomography (CT) as a curvilinear calcification along the posteroinferior rim of the glenoid.

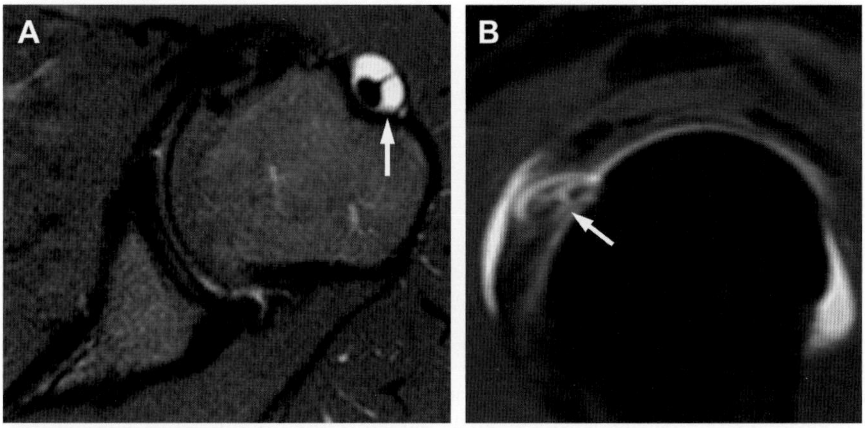

Fig. 7. Biceps lesions. (*A*) Fat-saturated proton-density (PD) axial MR image shows tenosynovitis with high signal fluid (*arrow*) surrounding the biceps tendon in the absence of a joint effusion. (*B*) Fat-saturated T1W coronal oblique MR image with intra-articular gadolinium shows gadolinium traversing the biceps tendon (*arrow*), compatible with a longitudinal split tear.

Anteroposterior radiographs of the shoulder do not routinely delineate the lesion, and an axillary or Stryker notch view is usually necessary for visualization.[77] MR imaging may show low signal intensity, corresponding to calcification, on T1W images (Fig. 8). A POLPSA lesion is an avulsion of the posterior capsule periosteum at its junction with the capsule and labrum, best seen on axial MR images (Fig. 9).[80]

BALL-THROWER'S FRACTURE

Spontaneous fractures of the humeral shaft may occur because of extreme muscular forces. Several cases have been reported while throwing an object such as a baseball, softball, cricket ball, or hand grenade.[81–84] The ball-thrower's fracture occurs mostly in people in their twenties who participate in overhead throwing at a recreational level, as it rarely occurs in competitive or professional athletes.[81] Recreational players are likely more susceptible to injury because they do not undergo protective adaptive changes such as muscular and cortical hypertrophy seen in professional athletes. The humeral shaft fracture probably occurs during the late cocking phase when the shoulder nears maximal external rotation whereby high torsional loads and shear forces may exceed the shear strength of bone, resulting in an external rotation spiral fracture (Fig. 10).[85] The majority of the fractures occur at the junction of the middle to distal thirds of the humerus, below the insertion of the deltoid muscle.[81] The ball-

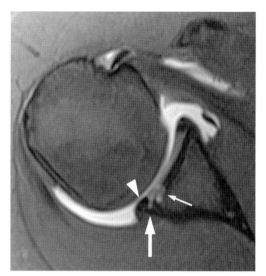

Fig. 9. POLPSA (posterior labrocapsular periosteal sleeve avulsion) lesion. Fat-saturated T1W axial MR image with intra-articular gadolinium shows avulsion of the posterior labrum (*arrowhead*) still attached to glenoid by intact sleeve of scapular periosteum (*large arrow*). Focal osteochondral defect is present at the chondrolabral junction (*small arrow*).

thrower's fracture may be complicated by radial nerve palsy, as the nerve may be lacerated or trapped at the intermuscular septum between the fracture fragments.[86]

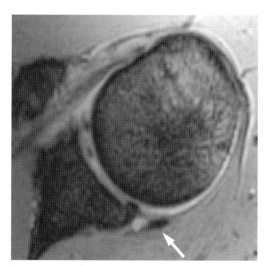

Fig. 8. Bennett lesion. Axial gradient-echo MR image shows curvilinear area of low signal intensity (*arrow*), corresponding to calcification, adjacent to the posterior inferior glenoid.

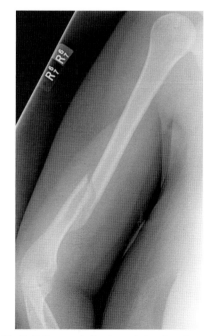

Fig. 10. Ball-thrower's fracture. Lateral radiograph of the humerus shows spiral fracture at the distal third of the humerus.

ELBOW INJURIES
Imaging of the Elbow

MR imaging is the preferred modality for evaluation of the soft tissues and ligaments of the elbow. Imaging may be performed with low–field-strength and high–field-strength systems, although there are limited clinical studies comparing their performance characteristics. The patient is ideally positioned supine with the elbow at the side; however, the patient may be scanned prone or on the side with the elbow extended as much as possible overhead. A dedicated surface coil centered at the olecranon is used to optimize SNR.

Axial images are obtained perpendicular to the humerus, and extend distally to include the radial tuberosity and biceps insertion. Coronal images are generated parallel to the epicondylar axis of the distal humerus on the axial plane while sagittal images are created perpendicular to the coronal plane. The standard unenhanced MR imaging protocol includes axial T1W, fat-saturated axial T2W, fat-saturated coronal PD, coronal short inversion-time inversion recovery (STIR), coronal T1W, sagittal STIR, and coronal 3-dimensional gradient-echo sequences.

Indications for direct MR arthrography of the throwing athlete's elbow include identification of UCL tears, loose bodies, synovial abnormalities, and assessing stability of an osteochondral injury.[87] Three sites may be used for joint puncture under fluoroscopic guidance: laterally into the radiocapitellar joint, posteriorly through the triceps, or posterolaterally between the humerus and olecranon.[88] The skin and soft tissues are anesthetized with 1% lidocaine. Up to 10 mL of a dilute gadolinium/iodinated contrast mixture is injected into the glenohumeral joint with a 22-gauge spinal needle. The standard direct MR arthrography protocol includes axial, coronal, and sagittal fat-saturated

T1W, coronal T2W, and fat-saturated coronal PD sequences.

Valgus Extension Overload

Valgus extension overload (VEO) is often seen in throwing athletes, and refers to impingement of the posteromedial olecranon tip against the medial wall of the olecranon fossa.[89] Large valgus stress with rapid elbow extension during the late cocking and early acceleration phases of overhead throwing produces lateral-compartment compressive forces and medial-compartment tensile forces. Repeated valgus loads during overhead throwing can lead to osteophyte formation on the posteromedial tip of the olecranon.[90] Osteophytes may fracture and form loose bodies within the joint.

Overhead-throwing athletes may experience posterior elbow pain at ball release when the elbow nears full extension.[91] Posteromedial impingement may be diagnosed clinically if the athlete's symptoms are reproduced with repeated valgus stress on the elbow at 20° to 30° of flexion while fully extending the elbow, known as a positive VEO test.[91] In a study of professional baseball players who underwent elbow surgery, posteromedial olecranon osteophytes were the most common diagnosis, affecting 65% of players.[92]

Initial evaluation for VEO is with anteroposterior, lateral, and oblique radiographs to evaluate for posteromedial olecranon osteophytes or loose bodies. Their absence does not exclude VEO, as clinical symptoms may be evident before osteophyte formation.[91] MR imaging may show a loss of focal cartilage along the ulnar or humeral articular surfaces, subchondral sclerosis, or subchondral edema, best seen on axial sequences (**Fig. 11**).[93] Injury to the UCL is also associated with posteromedial impingement.[94]

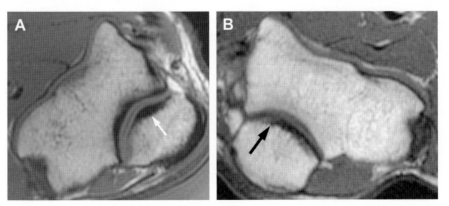

Fig. 11. Posteromedial impingement. (*A, B*) T1W axial MR image shows asymmetric subchondral sclerosis (*white arrow*) in the symptomatic throwing elbow compared with the asymptomatic nonthrowing elbow (*black arrow*).

Olecranon Stress Fractures

Repetitive abutment of the olecranon into the olecranon fossa or excessive tensile stress from the triceps tendon in throwing athletes may cause an olecranon stress fracture. Stress fractures result from insufficient bone remodeling in response to repetitive mechanical strain.[95]

Unlike VEO, clinical symptoms of an olecranon stress fracture often include posterolateral olecranon pain during and after throwing.[90] Pain with forced extension may also be seen, making it difficult to distinguish from VEO.[91]

Radiographs are the recommended initial test for elbow pain, although they are often normal when evaluating for stress fractures. MR imaging is helpful in identifying olecranon stress injuries before the development of a complete fracture. Stress fractures appear as linear decreased signal intensity on T1W images, typically with marrow edema, seen as increased signal intensity on fat-suppressed T2W or STIR images (**Fig. 12**).

Ulnar Collateral Ligament Injuries

The ulnar (or medial) collateral ligament (UCL) consists of the anterior bundle, the posterior bundle, and the transverse ligament. The anterior bundle of the UCL is the primary stabilizer of the elbow to valgus stress, particularly during the cocking and acceleration phase of throwing, and may be injured during repetitive throwing.[96,97] The anterior bundle originates from the anteroinferior aspect of the medial epicondyle and inserts on the sublime tubercle of the coronoid process (**Fig. 13**). The insertion site on the coronoid process may vary by up to 3 to 4 mm relative to the joint line as a normal variant, or secondary to age-related degenerative changes.[98] Underneath the UCL in normal elbows there is a thin layer of intra-articular fat, which may be effaced or absent with injury.[99]

UCL injury causes significant disability in the overhead-throwing athlete. Repetitive valgus stress leads to microtears, inflammation, and progressive laxity, with subsequent ligamentous tears. Athletes experience medial joint pain, occasionally with ulnar paresthesias, and usually notice a decrease in their pitching velocity and control.[100] The incidence of UCL injury has increased in baseball, particularly at the high school level. Risk factors in high school pitchers include overuse with an average of 8 months a year of competitive pitching, extensive off-season bullpen sessions, and high average pitch velocity.[100]

Radiographs are often the initial imaging study, although they cannot show direct ligamentous injury. However, heterotopic calcification in the region of the UCL, an indirect sign of injury, may be present in up to 93% of throwing athletes with elbow pain (**Fig. 14**).[101]

MR imaging is the preferred imaging modality for the evaluation of the UCL. Best seen on coronal images, the normal anterior band of the UCL has uniform low signal intensity on T1W and T2W images, although high–signal-intensity fat may interdigitate within the anterior bundle at its origin from the medial epicondyle.[98,102,103] A UCL sprain is characterized by increased ligamentous and periligamentous soft-tissue signal intensity, representing hemorrhage and edema, on T1W and T2W images.[104]

MR arthrography is much more sensitive (86%) than unenhanced MR imaging (14%) for the detection of partial-thickness tears of the UCL.[105,106] Partial-thickness tears are characterized by intraligamentous high signal intensity and discontinuity

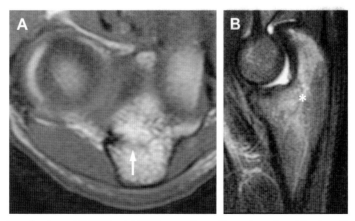

Fig. 12. Olecranon stress fracture. (*A*) T1W axial MR image shows linear low signal fracture line (*arrow*) traversing the olecranon. (*B*) Short inversion-time inversion recovery (STIR) sagittal MR image shows increased signal (*asterisk*), corresponding to marrow edema, in the olecranon.

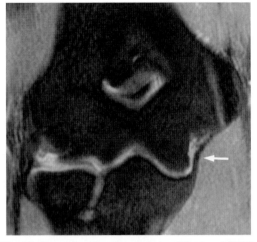

Fig. 13. Normal native ulnar collateral ligament (UCL). Fat-saturated PD coronal MR image shows normal low-signal anterior band of the UCL (*arrow*) extending from the inferior aspect of the medial epicondyle to the sublime tubercle.

or disruption of some fibers of the UCL (**Fig. 15**). Most tears occur within the midsubstance of the UCL, followed by tears at the distal attachment to the coronoid process and tears at the origin from the medial epicondyle.[97] Partial undersurface tearing of the anterior bundle of the UCL may show high signal or intra-articular contrast at the distal insertion near the sublime tubercle, often referred to as the "T-sign," which was originally described by CT arthrography.[106]

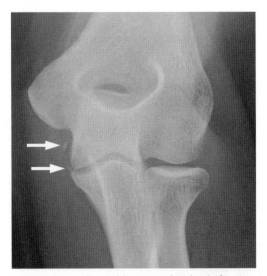

Fig. 14. Ulnar collateral ligament (UCL) calcifications. Anteroposterior (AP) radiograph of the elbow shows calcifications (*arrows*) in the distribution of the UCL, suggestive of chronic injury.

Unlike for the detection of partial-thickness tears, MR arthrography and unenhanced MR imaging are similarly sensitive (95%–100%) for the detection of full-thickness tears of the UCL.[105,106] Ligamentous discontinuity with possible retraction of the proximal and distal fibers is characteristic of full-thickness tears. Secondary findings include extravasation of joint effusion or contrast, in the case of direct arthrography, into the adjacent soft tissues (see **Fig. 15**).[107,108]

UCL reconstruction allows overhead-throwing athletes to return to their previous level of activity.[109] The UCL is typically repaired and sutured to an ipsilateral palmaris longus tendon graft secured with 1 ulnar tunnel and 2 medial epicondylar tunnels.[109] A normal taut UCL graft has a thickened appearance and variable MR signal intensity, with approximately 75% of grafts showing homogeneously low signal on T1W and T2W images (**Fig. 16**).[110] Findings of UCL graft degeneration include diffuse intermediate signal within an enlarged graft on T1W images with inability to discern graft fibers on T2W images.[110] MR arthrography is valuable for detecting UCL graft tears and shows gadolinium signal insinuating into the tear on T1W images and fluid signal intensity within the graft on T2W images.[110]

On rare occasions, avulsion fracture of the sublime tubercle may be a source of medial elbow pain in the overhead-throwing athlete. In one series of 8 patients, radiographs and MR imaging showed the avulsion fracture in 75% and 100% of athletes, respectively.[111] Avulsion fractures can occur with or without midsubstance tearing of the UCL, and differentiation is important because surgical fixation is different in each case.[111]

Ulnar Neuritis

Ulnar neuritis may occur at multiple anatomic sites along the course of the ulnar nerve. The overhead-throwing athlete is particularly vulnerable to compression and traction injury of the ulnar nerve at the cubital tunnel from repetitive valgus and extension forces. At the elbow, the ulnar nerve courses between the medial epicondyle and the olecranon and then enters the cubital tunnel, bound by the posterior band of the UCL laterally, the medial epicondylar groove anteriorly, and the arcuate ligament medially. Ulnar neuritis may also occur from compression from osteophytes, flexor muscle hypertrophy, or nerve subluxation.[90]

Clinical symptoms include medial elbow pain during overhead throwing with paresthesias in the ulnar forearm, ulnar hand, and ring and little fingers. Progressive symptoms may include pain

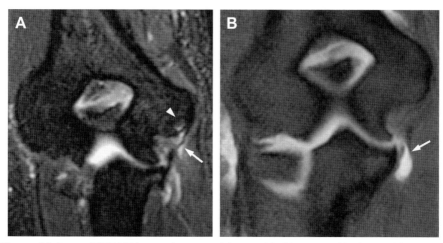

Fig. 15. UCL tear. (*A*) Coronal STIR MR image shows partial tear with thinning and high signal (*arrow*) of the proximal medial one-third of the anterior bundle of the UCL. Small focus of increased signal (*arrowhead*) within the adjacent medial epicondyle of the distal humerus represents a small cyst, likely from repetitive chronic trauma. (*B*) Fat-saturated T1W coronal MR image with intra-articular gadolinium shows focal disruption of the midsubstance of the anterior band of the UCL with extravasation of gadolinium into the medial soft tissues (*arrow*).

and paresthesias at rest, hand weakness, clumsy grip, and visible muscular atrophy.

MR imaging is effective in the evaluation of peripheral nerves and is based on the signal differences between the nerve and surrounding fat.[112] MR imaging has a very high sensitivity (>90%) for the diagnosis of ulnar nerve entrapment at the elbow.[113,114] The ulnar nerve is particularly conspicuous at the elbow because of surrounding fat and is best visualized on axial MR sequences with the elbow extended.[115] Normal nerves have a smooth round or ovoid shape, are isointense to muscle on T1W images, and are isointense or slightly hyperintense to muscle on T2W images.[112,115,116] Focal thickening with increased signal of the ulnar nerve on STIR or T2W images is

characteristic of ulnar neuropathy (**Fig. 17**). Chronic injury may lead to atrophy and fatty replacement of the innervated musculature, best seen on T1W images.[112]

Flexor-Pronator Muscle Group Injuries

The flexor-pronator group contains the musculotendinous structures of the medial elbow, with the pronator teres and flexor carpi radialis muscles most commonly injured.[117] Throwing athletes may develop a spectrum of injuries, commonly referred to as medial epicondylitis, ranging from acute or chronic tendinitis to acute muscle tears. Extreme valgus forces during the acceleration phase of throwing may exceed the tensile strength of the

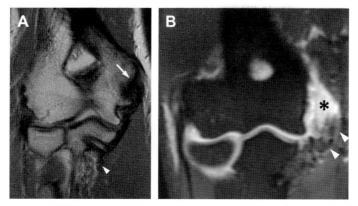

Fig. 16. UCL reconstruction. (*A*) PD coronal MR image shows normal UCL graft extending from humeral tunnel (*arrow*) to ulnar tunnel (*arrowhead*). (*B*) Fat-saturated T1W coronal MR image with intra-articular gadolinium shows full-thickness tear of UCL graft from humeral tunnel (*arrowheads*) and extravasation of gadolinium (*asterisk*).

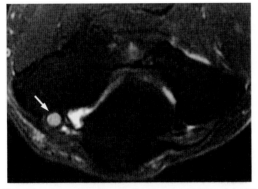

Fig. 17. Ulnar neuritis. Fat-saturated T2W axial MR image shows increased signal of an enlarged ulnar nerve (*arrow*) within the cubital tunnel.

medial musculotendinous and ligamentous structures, first in the flexor-pronator muscle group and then the deeper UCL.[117] Thus the primary differential diagnosis of medial epicondylitis includes injury to the UCL.

Physical examination findings include medial elbow pain worsened by resistance to forearm pronation, and wrist flexion and tenderness to palpation over the pronator teres and flexor carpi ulnaris muscles. Medial epicondylitis is initially treated with active rest, anti-inflammatory medication, physical therapy, and gradual return to overhead throwing. Surgical treatment is usually recommended if there is no response to 3 to 6 months of nonoperative management or if imaging indicates tendon disruption.[117]

The most common MR finding of medial epicondylitis is increased signal intensity within the common flexor tendon on both T1W and T2W images, best seen on axial and coronal sequences.[118] However, abnormal signal within

the common flexor tendon may also be seen in asymptomatic individuals, indicating normal degenerative changes within the tendon.[118] The most specific findings of medial epicondylitis include intermediate to high signal intensity within the common flexor tendon with paratendinous soft-tissue edema (**Fig. 18**).[118] Possible additional findings include bone marrow edema of the medial epicondyle and tears of the anterior bundle of the UCL.

PEDIATRIC INJURIES
Medial Epicondylar Apophysitis

Medial elbow pain and soreness is very common among Little League baseball players, affecting up to 58% of pitchers, 63% of catchers, and 47% of fielders.[119–121] The apophysis is a biomechanical weak link in the skeletally immature elbow, caused by hormonal factors and thinning of the ring of Ranvier (chondrocytes integral for growth plate expansion) during puberty.[122] Little League elbow classically refers to medial epicondylar apophysitis, an overuse traction injury to the medial epicondylar apophysis.[123] Unlike in the adult overhead thrower, the UCL is much stronger than the medial epicondyle apophyseal growth plate. Extreme valgus position of the elbow during the late cocking and early acceleration phase of throwing places excessive traction load on the weak epicondyle apophyseal growth plate from both the UCL and forearm flexor-pronator musculature.[90,124]

Clinical symptoms include medial elbow soreness during or after throwing, without signs of instability with valgus stress testing of the elbow.[121,125] Management includes initial treatment with ice and nonsteroidal anti-inflammatories, cessation of pitching for 4 to 6 weeks, and physical therapy.[90]

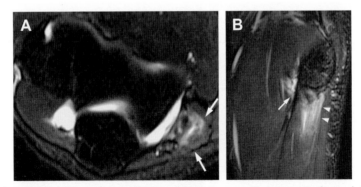

Fig. 18. Medial epicondylitis. (*A*) Fat-saturated T2W axial MR image with intra-articular gadolinium shows paratendinous high signal (*arrows*) of the common flexor tendon origin. (*B*) Fat-saturated T2W sagittal MR image with intra-articular gadolinium shows high signal in the margin of the pronator teres muscle adjacent to the common flexor tendon (*arrow*) and flexor digitorum superficialis muscle (*arrowheads*), compatible with medial epicondylitis.

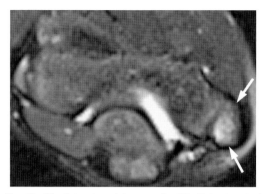

Fig. 19. Medial epicondylar apophysitis. Fat-saturated T2W axial MR image shows increased signal (*arrows*) in the apophysis of the medial epicondyle, compatible with medial epicondylar apophysitis.

Radiographs may show medial epicondylar apophysis hypertrophy, fragmentation, or apophysis separation from the medial humeral metaphysis of greater than 1 mm.[121] Contralateral comparison views may be helpful in detecting subtle apophysis asymmetry or irregularity. MR imaging findings include edema in the medial epicondylar apophysis and/or medial humeral metaphysis on fat-saturated T2W or STIR images (**Fig. 19**). Muscular edema and tendinopathy may also affect the common flexor tendon.[125] Similar to radiographs, separation and widening of more than 1 mm between the apophysis and humeral metaphysis may be seen on coronal sequences.[125] The UCL has a normal appearance without evidence of attenuation or tearing.[125] Although MR imaging is more sensitive than radiographs for the evaluation of Little League elbow, the additional imaging findings do not change clinical management.[125]

Medial Epicondyle Avulsion

Medial epicondyle avulsion is typically an acute injury that occurs with a single pitch in the overhead-throwing athlete, and there may be an associated "pop" or "crack" with an inability to continue pitching.[122,126,127] The avulsion typically occurs during the late cocking or early acceleration phase of throwing, and is due to acute overload failure of the medial epicondyle from valgus stress and flexor-pronator muscle group contraction.[122] Woods and Tullos[127] have classified medial epicondyle avulsions into 3 types, based on the age of the patient and size of fragment. Type 1 lesions involve the entire medial epicondyle, which is often displaced and rotated, in athletes aged 14 years or younger.[127] Type 2 and 3 lesions occur after medial epicondyle fusion in athletes aged 15 years or older: type 2 lesions involve a large medial epicondyle avulsion with or without UCL injury, and type 3 lesions involve a small medial epicondyle avulsion typically with a tear of the midportion of the anterior band of the UCL (**Fig. 20**).[127]

Osteochondral Defect of the Capitellum

Osteochondral defect, or osteochondral dissecans (OCD), is a noninflammatory degeneration of subchondral bone thought to be due to repetitive compressive forces, often seen with overhead throwing in adolescents.[128,129] OCD of the elbow occurs mostly commonly in the capitellum, although it may also occur in the trochlea, radial head, olecranon, and olecranon fossa.[130–132] High valgus forces across the elbow during the late cocking and early acceleration phases of throwing cause significant compression to the lateral radiocapitellar joint. Repetitive radiocapitellar

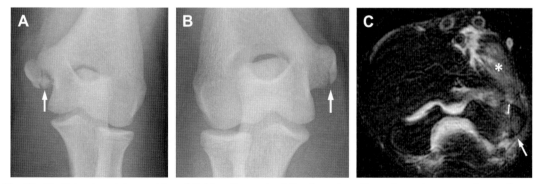

Fig. 20. Medial epicondylar avulsion. (*A*) AP radiograph of the throwing elbow shows fragmentation and separation of the medial epicondyle (*arrow*), suggestive of an avulsion fracture. (*B*) AP radiograph of the nonthrowing elbow shows normal morphology of the medial epicondyle (*arrow*). (*C*) Fat-saturated T2W axial MR image in a different patient shows avulsion fracture of medial epicondyle (*arrow*) with anterior displacement (*double-headed arrow*) of the apophysis. Increased signal (*asterisk*) within the pronator teres muscle indicates a strain.

compression on an immature epiphysis can lead to subchondral flattening and, ultimately, breakdown and fragmentation of articular cartilage and subchondral bone.[133]

Clinical symptoms include lateral elbow pain that is insidious in onset, progressive, and often relieved by rest. The most common physical finding is tenderness over the radiocapitellar joint and reproducible pain during the radiocapitellar compression test, which involves active forearm pronation and supination at full elbow extension.[133,134]

Radiographs of the elbow are often the initial imaging study for the evaluation of suspected OCD. Radiographs in the early stages of OCD of the capitellum may be normal. In later stages of OCD, the capitellum may show flattening of its contour, focal rarefaction, nondisplaced fragmentation, and possibly focal articular defect and loose body formation.[135,136]

MR imaging has superior sensitivity to radiography for the early detection of OCD of the capitellum.[137,138] OCD of the capitellum involves the anterolateral aspect of the capitellum, and is best seen on T1W images (Fig. 21).[139] This feature should not be mistaken for the normal pseudodefect of the capitellum, which is along the posteroinferior aspect of the capitellum and the nonarticular surface of the lateral epicondyle

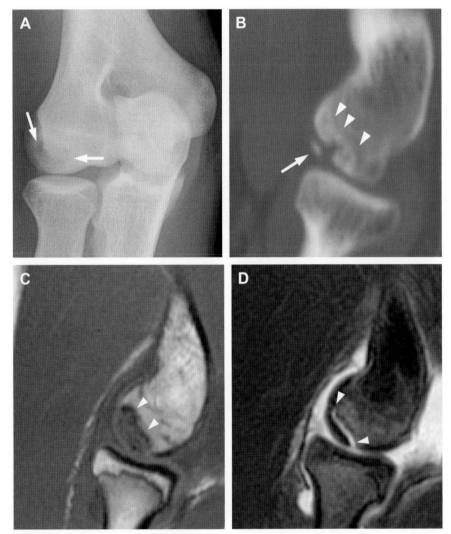

Fig. 21. Osteochondral dissecans (OCD) of capitellum. (A) Oblique radiograph of the elbow shows ovoid lucency (arrows) in the capitellum, compatible with OCD. (B) Sagittal reformatted CT image in another patient shows sclerosis and cortical irregularity (arrowheads) of the anterolateral capitellum with adjacent loose body (arrow). (C, D) Sagittal T1W MR image (C) in a different patient shows low-signal fragment (arrowheads) in the anterolateral capitellum while a sagittal T2W MR image (D) shows high-signal fluid (arrowheads) extending between the base of the fragment and humerus, indicating fragment instability.

(see **Fig. 21**).[140] Stable and unstable OCD lesions may be differentiated on T2W images, as they have different signal characteristics at the periphery of the lesion. Unstable OCD of the capitellum shows a peripheral ring of high signal intensity and/or underlying fluid-filled cysts (see **Fig. 21**), whereas stable OCD lesions show peripheral low signal intensity.[139] After intravenous gadolinium contrast, enhancement of the OCD lesion suggests viability with an intact vascular supply.[141] However, diffuse enhancement at the capitellar fragment and subchondral bone interface suggests reparative granulation tissue and fragment instability.[142]

SUMMARY

The throwing athlete is at risk for a wide range of abnormalities to the shoulder and elbow from extreme ranges of motion and stress during the various phases of throwing. An understanding of the throwing motion and the various injuries that occur during each phase allows for improved detection of these injuries on imaging studies. MR imaging is excellent at characterization of ligamentous, tendinous, and osseous abnormalities of the shoulder and elbow, and, when combined with a clinical examination, usually tailors appropriate treatment for the athlete so that he or she may return to competition.

REFERENCES

1. Waris W. Elbow injuries of javelin-throwers. Acta chir Scand 1946;93(6):563–75.
2. Dillman CJ, Fleisig GS, Andrews JR. Biomechanics of pitching with emphasis upon shoulder kinematics. J Orthop Sports Phys Ther 1993;18(2):402–8.
3. Meister K. Injuries to the shoulder in the throwing athlete. Part one: biomechanics/pathophysiology/classification of injury. Am J Sports Med 2000; 28(2):265–75.
4. Werner SL, Fleisig GS, Dillman CJ, et al. Biomechanics of the elbow during baseball pitching. J Orthop Sports Phys Ther 1993;17(6):274–8.
5. Park SS, Loebenberg ML, Rokito AS, et al. The shoulder in baseball pitching: biomechanics and related injuries—part 1. Bull Hosp Jt Dis 2002; 61(1–2):68–79.
6. Jobe FW, Moynes DR, Tibone JE, et al. An EMG analysis of the shoulder in pitching. A second report. Am J Sports Med 1984;12(3):218–20.
7. Altchek DW, Dines DM. Shoulder injuries in the throwing athlete. J Am Acad Orthop Surg 1995; 3(3):159–65.
8. Fleisig GS, Barrentine SW, Zheng N, et al. Kinematic and kinetic comparison of baseball pitching among various levels of development. J Biomech 1999;32(12):1371–5.
9. Sabick MB, Torry MR, Lawton RL, et al. Valgus torque in youth baseball pitchers: a biomechanical study. J Shoulder Elbow Surg 2004;13(3):349–55.
10. Harryman DT 2nd, Sidles JA, Clark JM, et al. Translation of the humeral head on the glenoid with passive glenohumeral motion. J Bone Joint Surg Am 1990;72(9):1334–43.
11. Morrey BF, An KN. Articular and ligamentous contributions to the stability of the elbow joint. Am J Sports Med 1983;11(5):315–9.
12. Fleisig GS, Andrews JR, Dillman CJ, et al. Kinetics of baseball pitching with implications about injury mechanisms. Am J Sports Med 1995;23(2):233–9.
13. Gainor BJ, Piotrowski G, Puhl J, et al. The throw: biomechanics and acute injury. Am J Sports Med 1980;8(2):114–8.
14. Lintner D, Noonan TJ, Kibler WB. Injury patterns and biomechanics of the athlete's shoulder. Clin Sports Med 2008;27(4):527–51.
15. Tung GA, Entzian D, Green A, et al. High-field and low-field MR imaging of superior glenoid labral tears and associated tendon injuries. AJR Am J Roentgenol 2000;174(4):1107–14.
16. Magee T, Shapiro M, Williams D. Comparison of high-field-strength versus low-field-strength MRI of the shoulder. AJR Am J Roentgenol 2003; 181(5):1211–5.
17. Shellock FG, Bert JM, Fritts HM, et al. Evaluation of the rotator cuff and glenoid labrum using a 0.2-Tesla extremity magnetic resonance (MR) system: MR results compared to surgical findings. J Magn Reson Imaging 2001;14(6): 763–70.
18. Allmann KH, Walter O, Laubenberger J, et al. Magnetic resonance diagnosis of the anterior labrum and capsule. Effect of field strength on efficacy. Invest Radiol 1998;33(7):415–20.
19. Davis SJ, Teresi LM, Bradley WG, et al. Effect of arm rotation on MR imaging of the rotator cuff. Radiology 1991;181(1):265–8.
20. Kwak SM, Brown RR, Trudell D, et al. Glenohumeral joint: comparison of shoulder positions at MR arthrography. Radiology 1998;208(2):375–80.
21. Lee SY, Lee JK. Horizontal component of partial-thickness tears of rotator cuff: imaging characteristics and comparison of ABER view with oblique coronal view at MR arthrography initial results. Radiology 2002;224(2):470–6.
22. Tirman PF, Bost FW, Steinbach LS, et al. MR arthrographic depiction of tears of the rotator cuff: benefit of abduction and external rotation of the arm. Radiology 1994;192(3):851–6.
23. Cvitanic O, Tirman PF, Feller JF, et al. Using abduction and external rotation of the shoulder to increase the sensitivity of MR arthrography in

revealing tears of the anterior glenoid labrum. AJR Am J Roentgenol 1997;169(3):837–44.

24. Saleem AM, Lee JK, Novak LM. Usefulness of the abduction and external rotation views in shoulder MR arthrography. AJR Am J Roentgenol 2008; 191(4):1024–30.

25. Park SS, Loebenberg ML, Rokito AS, et al. The shoulder in baseball pitching: biomechanics and related injuries-part 2. Bull Hosp Jt Dis 2002; 61(1–2):80–8.

26. de Jesus JO, Parker L, Frangos AJ, et al. Accuracy of MRI, MR arthrography, and ultrasound in the diagnosis of rotator cuff tears: a meta-analysis. AJR Am J Roentgenol 2009;192(6): 1701–7.

27. Ellman H. Diagnosis and treatment of incomplete rotator cuff tears. Clin Orthop Relat Res 1990;(254): 64–74.

28. Ellman H. Arthroscopic subacromial decompression: analysis of one- to three-year results. Arthroscopy 1987;3(3):173–81.

29. Uhthoff HK, Sano H. Pathology of failure of the rotator cuff tendon. Orthop Clin North Am 1997; 28(1):31–41.

30. Vinson EN, Helms CA, Higgins LD. Rim-rent tear of the rotator cuff: a common and easily overlooked partial tear. AJR Am J Roentgenol 2007;189(4): 943–6.

31. Tuite MJ, Turnbull JR, Orwin JF. Anterior versus posterior, and rim-rent rotator cuff tears: prevalence and MR sensitivity. Skeletal Radiol 1998; 27(5):237–43.

32. Millstein ES, Snyder SJ. Arthroscopic management of partial, full-thickness, and complex rotator cuff tears: indications, techniques, and complications. Arthroscopy 2003;19(Suppl 1):189–99.

33. Tuite MJ. MR imaging of sports injuries to the rotator cuff. Magn Reson Imaging Clin N Am 2003;11(2):207–19, v.

34. Conway JE. Arthroscopic repair of partial-thickness rotator cuff tears and SLAP lesions in professional baseball players. Orthop Clin North Am 2001; 32(3):443–56.

35. Jobe FW, Kvitne RS, Giangarra CE. Shoulder pain in the overhand or throwing athlete. The relationship of anterior instability and rotator cuff impingement. Orthop Rev 1989;18(9):963–75.

36. Bigliani LU, Morrison DS, April EW. The morphology of the acromion and its relationship to rotator cuff tears. Orthop Trans 1986;10:228.

37. Park JG, Lee JK, Phelps CT. Os acromiale associated with rotator cuff impingement: MR imaging of the shoulder. Radiology 1994;193(1):255–7.

38. Cowderoy GA, Lisle DA, O'Connell PT. Overuse and impingement syndromes of the shoulder in the athlete. Magn Reson Imaging Clin N Am 2009;17(4):577–93, v.

39. Ouellette H, Labis J, Bredella M, et al. Spectrum of shoulder injuries in the baseball pitcher. Skeletal Radiol 2008;37(6):491–8.

40. Halbrecht JL, Tirman P, Atkin D. Internal impingement of the shoulder: comparison of findings between the throwing and nonthrowing shoulders of college baseball players. Arthroscopy 1999; 15(3):253–8.

41. Bergin D. Imaging shoulder instability in the athlete. Magn Reson Imaging Clin N Am 2009; 17(4):595–615, v.

42. Burkhart SS, Morgan CD, Kibler WB. The disabled throwing shoulder: spectrum of pathology Part I: pathoanatomy and biomechanics. Arthroscopy 2003;19(4):404–20.

43. Greiwe RM, Ahmad CS. Management of the throwing shoulder: cuff, labrum and internal impingement. Orthop Clin North Am 2010;41(3): 309–23.

44. Moosikasuwan JB, Miller TT, Dines DM. Imaging of the painful shoulder in throwing athletes. Clin Sports Med 2006;25(3):433–43, vi.

45. Tirman PF, Bost FW, Garvin GJ, et al. Posterosuperior glenoid impingement of the shoulder: findings at MR imaging and MR arthrography with arthroscopic correlation. Radiology 1994;193(2): 431–6.

46. Tirman PF, Applegate GR, Flannigan BD, et al. Magnetic resonance arthrography of the shoulder. Magn Reson Imaging Clin N Am 1993; 1(1):125–42.

47. Flannigan B, Kursunoglu-Brahme S, Snyder S, et al. MR arthrography of the shoulder: comparison with conventional MR imaging. AJR Am J Roentgenol 1990;155(4):829–32.

48. Giaroli EL, Major NM, Higgins LD. MRI of internal impingement of the shoulder. AJR Am J Roentgenol 2005;185(4):925–9.

49. Dines DM, Warren RF, Inglis AE, et al. The coracoid impingement syndrome. J Bone Joint Surg Br 1990;72(2):314–6.

50. Paulson MM, Watnik NF, Dines DM. Coracoid impingement syndrome, rotator interval reconstruction, and biceps tenodesis in the overhead athlete. Orthop Clin North Am 2001;32(3):485–93, ix.

51. Kragh JF Jr, Doukas WC, Basamania CJ. Primary coracoid impingement syndrome. Am J Orthop (Belle Mead NJ) 2004;33(5):229–32 [discussion: 232].

52. Giaroli EL, Major NM, Lemley DE, et al. Coracohumeral interval imaging in subcoracoid impingement syndrome on MRI. AJR Am J Roentgenol 2006;186(1):242–6.

53. Lo IK, Burkhart SS. The etiology and assessment of subscapularis tendon tears: a case for subcoracoid impingement, the roller-wringer effect, and TUFF lesions of the subscapularis. Arthroscopy 2003;19(10):1142–50.

54. Habermeyer P, Schuller U, Wiedemann E. The intra-articular pressure of the shoulder: an experimental study on the role of the glenoid labrum in stabilizing the joint. Arthroscopy 1992;8(2): 166–72.

55. Fehringer EV, Schmidt GR, Boorman RS, et al. The anteroinferior labrum helps center the humeral head on the glenoid. J Shoulder Elbow Surg 2003;12(1):53–8.

56. Andrews JR, Carson WG Jr, McLeod WD. Glenoid labrum tears related to the long head of the biceps. Am J Sports Med 1985;13(5):337–41.

57. Snyder SJ, Karzel RP, Del Pizzo W, et al. SLAP lesions of the shoulder. Arthroscopy 1990;6(4):274–9.

58. Maffet MW, Gartsman GM, Moseley B. Superior labrum-biceps tendon complex lesions of the shoulder. Am J Sports Med 1995;23(1):93–8.

59. Morgan CD, Burkhart SS, Palmeri M, et al. Type II SLAP lesions: three subtypes and their relationships to superior instability and rotator cuff tears. Arthroscopy 1998;14(6):553–65.

60. Powell SE, Nord KD, Ryu RK. Diagnosis, classification and treatment of SLAP lesions. Oper Tech Sports Med 2004;12:99–110.

61. Abrams GD, Safran MR. Diagnosis and management of superior labrum anterior posterior lesions in overhead athletes. Br J Sports Med 2010;44(5):311–8.

62. Mileski RA, Snyder SJ. Superior labral lesions in the shoulder: pathoanatomy and surgical management. J Am Acad Orthop Surg 1998;6(2):121–31.

63. Jin W, Ryu KN, Kwon SH, et al. MR arthrography in the differential diagnosis of type II superior labral anteroposterior lesion and sublabral recess. AJR Am J Roentgenol 2006;187(4):887–93.

64. Kuhn JE, Lindholm SR, Huston LJ, et al. Failure of the biceps superior labral complex: a cadaveric biomechanical investigation comparing the late cocking and early deceleration positions of throwing. Arthroscopy 2003;19(4):373–9.

65. Yeh ML, Lintner D, Luo ZP. Stress distribution in the superior labrum during throwing motion. Am J Sports Med 2005;33(3):395–401.

66. Burkhart SS, Morgan CD. The peel-back mechanism: its role in producing and extending posterior type II SLAP lesions and its effect on SLAP repair rehabilitation. Arthroscopy 1998;14(6):637–40.

67. Bedi A, Allen AA. Superior labral lesions anterior to posterior-evaluation and arthroscopic management. Clin Sports Med 2008;27(4):607–30.

68. Tuite MJ, Cirillo RL, De Smet AA, et al. Superior labrum anterior-posterior (SLAP) tears: evaluation of three MR signs on T2-weighted images. Radiology 2000;215(3):841–5.

69. Rodosky MW, Harner CD, Fu FH. The role of the long head of the biceps muscle and superior glenoid labrum in anterior stability of the shoulder. Am J Sports Med 1994;22(1):121–30.

70. Post M, Benca P. Primary tendinitis of the long head of the biceps. Clin Orthop Relat Res 1989;(246): 117–25.

71. Ahrens PM, Boileau P. The long head of biceps and associated tendinopathy. J Bone Joint Surg Br 2007;89(8):1001–9.

72. Tuckman GA. Abnormalities of the long head of the biceps tendon of the shoulder: MR imaging findings. AJR Am J Roentgenol 1994;163(5):1183–8.

73. Kaplan PA, Bryans KC, Davick JP, et al. MR imaging of the normal shoulder: variants and pitfalls. Radiology 1992;184(2):519–24.

74. Beall DP, Williamson EE, Ly JQ, et al. Association of biceps tendon tears with rotator cuff abnormalities: degree of correlation with tears of the anterior and superior portions of the rotator cuff. AJR Am J Roentgenol 2003;180(3):633–9.

75. Chan TW, Dalinka MK, Kneeland JB, et al. Biceps tendon dislocation: evaluation with MR imaging. Radiology 1991;179(3):649–52.

76. Ferrari JD, Ferrari DA, Coumas J, et al. Posterior ossification of the shoulder: the Bennett lesion. Etiology, diagnosis, and treatment. Am J Sports Med 1994;22(2):171–5 [discussion: 175–6].

77. Wright RW, Paletta GA Jr. Prevalence of the Bennett lesion of the shoulder in major league pitchers. Am J Sports Med 2004;32(1):121–4.

78. De Maeseneer M, Jaovisidha S, Jacobson JA, et al. The Bennett lesion of the shoulder. J Comput Assist Tomogr 1998;22(1):31–4.

79. Shah N, Tung GA. Imaging signs of posterior glenohumeral instability. AJR Am J Roentgenol 2009; 192(3):730–5.

80. Yu JS, Ashman CJ, Jones G. The POLPSA lesion: MR imaging findings with arthroscopic correlation in patients with posterior instability. Skeletal Radiol 2002;31(7):396–9.

81. Ogawa K, Yoshida A. Throwing fracture of the humeral shaft. An analysis of 90 patients. Am J Sports Med 1998;26(2):242–6.

82. Curtin P, Taylor C, Rice J. Thrower's fracture of the humerus with radial nerve palsy: an unfamiliar softball injury. Br J Sports Med 2005;39(11):e40.

83. Kaplan H, Kiral A, Kuskucu M, et al. Report of eight cases of humeral fracture following the throwing of hand grenades. Arch Orthop Trauma Surg 1998; 117(1–2):50–2.

84. Evans PA, Farnell RD, Moalypour S, et al. Thrower's fracture: a comparison of two presentations of a rare fracture. J Accid Emerg Med 1995;12(3): 222–4.

85. Sabick MB, Torry MR, Kim YK, et al. Humeral torque in professional baseball pitchers. Am J Sports Med 2004;32(4):892–8.

86. Holstein A, Lewis GM. Fractures of the humerus with radial-nerve paralysis. J Bone Joint Surg Am 1963;45:1382–8.

87. Steinbach LS, Schwartz M. Elbow arthrography. Radiol Clin North Am 1998;36(4):635–49.

88. Chundru U, Riley GM, Steinbach LS. Magnetic resonance arthrography. Radiol Clin North Am 2009;47(3):471–94.

89. Wilson FD, Andrews JR, Blackburn TA, et al. Valgus extension overload in the pitching elbow. Am J Sports Med 1983;11(2):83–8.

90. Cain EL Jr, Dugas JR, Wolf RS, et al. Elbow injuries in throwing athletes: a current concepts review. Am J Sports Med 2003;31(4):621–35.

91. Dugas JR. Valgus extension overload: diagnosis and treatment. Clin Sports Med 2010; 29(4):645–54.

92. Andrews JR, Timmerman LA. Outcome of elbow surgery in professional baseball players. Am J Sports Med 1995;23(4):407–13.

93. Anderson MW, Alford BA. Overhead throwing injuries of the shoulder and elbow. Radiol Clin North Am 2010;48(6):1137–54.

94. Kooima CL, Anderson K, Craig JV, et al. Evidence of subclinical medial collateral ligament injury and posteromedial impingement in professional baseball players. Am J Sports Med 2004;32(7):1602–6.

95. Bennell KL, Malcolm SA, Wark JD, et al. Models for the pathogenesis of stress fractures in athletes. Br J Sports Med 1996;30(3):200–4.

96. Davidson PA, Pink M, Perry J, et al. Functional anatomy of the flexor pronator muscle group in relation to the medial collateral ligament of the elbow. Am J Sports Med 1995;23(2):245–50.

97. Conway JE, Jobe FW, Glousman RE, et al. Medial instability of the elbow in throwing athletes. Treatment by repair or reconstruction of the ulnar collateral ligament. J Bone Joint Surg Am 1992;74(1): 67–83.

98. Munshi M, Pretterklieber ML, Chung CB, et al. Anterior bundle of ulnar collateral ligament: evaluation of anatomic relationships by using MR imaging, MR arthrography, and gross anatomic and histologic analysis. Radiology 2004;231(3): 797–803.

99. Sugimoto H, Ohsawa T. Ulnar collateral ligament in the growing elbow: MR imaging of normal development and throwing injuries. Radiology 1994;192(2): 417–22.

100. Petty DH, Andrews JR, Fleisig GS, et al. Ulnar collateral ligament reconstruction in high school baseball players: clinical results and injury risk factors. Am J Sports Med 2004;32(5):1158–64.

101. Mulligan SA, Schwartz ML, Broussard MF, et al. Heterotopic calcification and tears of the ulnar collateral ligament: radiographic and MR imaging findings. AJR Am J Roentgenol 2000;175(4):1099–102.

102. Mirowitz SA, London SL. Ulnar collateral ligament injury in baseball pitchers: MR imaging evaluation. Radiology 1992;185(2):573–6.

103. Nakanishi K, Masatomi T, Ochi T, et al. MR arthrography of elbow: evaluation of the ulnar collateral ligament of elbow. Skeletal Radiol 1996;25(7):629–34.

104. Patten RM. Overuse syndromes and injuries involving the elbow: MR imaging findings. AJR Am J Roentgenol 1995;164(5):1205–11.

105. Schwartz ML, al-Zahrani S, Morwessel RM, et al. Ulnar collateral ligament injury in the throwing athlete: evaluation with saline-enhanced MR arthrography. Radiology 1995;197(1):297–9.

106. Timmerman LA, Schwartz ML, Andrews JR. Preoperative evaluation of the ulnar collateral ligament by magnetic resonance imaging and computed tomography arthrography. Evaluation in 25 baseball players with surgical confirmation. Am J Sports Med 1994;22(1):26–31 [discussion: 32].

107. Sugimoto H, Hyodoh K, Shinozaki T. Throwing injury of the elbow: assessment with gradient three-dimensional, Fourier transform gradient-echo and short tau inversion recovery images. J Magn Reson Imaging 1998;8(2):487–92.

108. Cotten A, Jacobson J, Brossmann J, et al. Collateral ligaments of the elbow: conventional MR imaging and MR arthrography with coronal oblique plane and elbow flexion. Radiology 1997;204(3):806–12.

109. Cain EL Jr, Andrews JR, Dugas JR, et al. Outcome of ulnar collateral ligament reconstruction of the elbow in 1281 athletes: results in 743 athletes with minimum 2-year follow-up. Am J Sports Med 2010;38(12):2426–34.

110. Wear SA, Thornton DD, Schwartz ML, et al. MRI of the reconstructed ulnar collateral ligament. AJR Am J Roentgenol 2011;197(5):1198–204.

111. Salvo JP, Rizio L 3rd, Zvijac JE, et al. Avulsion fracture of the ulnar sublime tubercle in overhead throwing athletes. Am J Sports Med 2002;30(3):426–31.

112. Bordalo-Rodrigues M, Rosenberg ZS. MR imaging of entrapment neuropathies at the elbow. Magn Reson Imaging Clin N Am 2004;12(2):247–63, vi.

113. Britz GW, Haynor DR, Kuntz C, et al. Ulnar nerve entrapment at the elbow: correlation of magnetic resonance imaging, clinical, electrodiagnostic, and intraoperative findings. Neurosurgery 1996; 38(3):458–65 [discussion: 465].

114. Vucic S, Cordato DJ, Yiannikas C, et al. Utility of magnetic resonance imaging in diagnosing ulnar neuropathy at the elbow. Clin Neurophysiol 2006; 117(3):590–5.

115. Rosenberg ZS, Beltran J, Cheung YY, et al. The elbow: MR features of nerve disorders. Radiology 1993;188(1):235–40.

116. Rosenberg ZS, Bencardino J, Beltran J. MR features of nerve disorders at the elbow. Magn Reson Imaging Clin N Am 1997;5(3):545–65.

117. Ciccotti MC, Schwartz MA, Ciccotti MG. Diagnosis and treatment of medial epicondylitis of the elbow. Clin Sports Med 2004;23(4):693–705, xi.

118. Kijowski R, De Smet AA. Magnetic resonance imaging findings in patients with medial epicondylitis. Skeletal Radiol 2005;34(4):196–202.

119. Gugenheim JJ Jr, Stanley RF, Woods GW, et al. Little League survey: the Houston study. Am J Sports Med 1976;4(5):189–200.

120. Larson RL, Singer KM, Bergstrom R, et al. Little League survey: the Eugene study. Am J Sports Med 1976;4(5):201–9.

121. Hang DW, Chao CM, Hang YS. A clinical and roentgenographic study of Little League elbow. Am J Sports Med 2004;32(1):79–84.

122. Hughes PE, Paletta GA. Little Leaguer's elbow, medial epicondyle injury, and osteochondritis dissecans. Sports Med Arthrosc 2003;11(1):30–9.

123. Brogdon BG, Crow NE. Little Leaguer's elbow. Am J Roentgenol Radium Ther Nucl Med 1960;83:671–5.

124. Greiwe RM, Saifi C, Ahmad CS. Pediatric sports elbow injuries. Clin Sports Med 2010;29(4):677–703.

125. Wei AS, Khana S, Limpisvasti O, et al. Clinical and magnetic resonance imaging findings associated with Little League elbow. J Pediatr Orthop 2010; 30(7):715–9.

126. Case SL, Hennrikus WL. Surgical treatment of displaced medial epicondyle fractures in adolescent athletes. Am J Sports Med 1997;25(5):682–6.

127. Woods GW, Tullos HS. Elbow instability and medial epicondyle fractures. Am J Sports Med 1977;5(1):23–30.

128. Lord J, Winell JJ. Overuse injuries in pediatric athletes. Curr Opin Pediatr 2004;16(1):47–50.

129. Lyman S, Fleisig GS, Waterbor JW, et al. Longitudinal study of elbow and shoulder pain in youth baseball pitchers. Med Sci Sports Exerc 2001; 33(11):1803–10.

130. Joji S, Murakami T, Murao T. Osteochondritis dissecans developing in the trochlea humeri: a case report. J Shoulder Elbow Surg 2001; 10(3):295–7.

131. Dotzis A, Galissier B, Peyrou P, et al. Osteochondritis dissecans of the radial head: a case report. J Shoulder Elbow Surg 2009;18(1):e18–21.

132. Stubbs MJ, Field LD, Savoie FH 3rd. Osteochondritis dissecans of the elbow. Clin Sports Med 2001; 20(1):1–9.

133. Baker CL 3rd, Romeo AA, Baker CL Jr. Osteochondritis dissecans of the capitellum. Am J Sports Med 2010;38(9):1917–28.

134. McManama GB Jr, Micheli LJ, Berry MV, et al. The surgical treatment of osteochondritis of the capitellum. Am J Sports Med 1985;13(1):11–21.

135. Kijowski R, De Smet AA. Radiography of the elbow for evaluation of patients with osteochondritis dissecans of the capitellum. Skeletal Radiol 2005; 34(5):266–71.

136. Takahara M, Ogino T, Takagi M, et al. Natural progression of osteochondritis dissecans of the humeral capitellum: initial observations. Radiology 2000;216(1):207–12.

137. Takahara M, Shundo M, Kondo M, et al. Early detection of osteochondritis dissecans of the capitellum in young baseball players. Report of three cases. J Bone Joint Surg Am 1998;80(6):892–7.

138. Janarv PM, Hesser U, Hirsch G. Osteochondral lesions in the radiocapitellar joint in the skeletally immature: radiographic, MRI, and arthroscopic findings in 13 consecutive cases. J Pediatr Orthop 1997;17(3):311–4.

139. Kijowski R, De Smet AA. MRI findings of osteochondritis dissecans of the capitellum with surgical correlation. AJR Am J Roentgenol 2005;185(6): 1453–9.

140. Rosenberg ZS, Beltran J, Cheung YY. Pseudodefect of the capitellum: potential MR imaging pitfall. Radiology 1994;191(3):821–3.

141. Kijowski R, Tuite M, Sanford M. Magnetic resonance imaging of the elbow. Part I: normal anatomy, imaging technique, and osseous abnormalities. Skeletal Radiol 2004;33(12):685–97.

142. Peiss J, Adam G, Casser R, et al. Gadopentate-dimeglumine-enhanced MR imaging of osteonecrosis and osteochondritis dissecans of the elbow: initial experience. Skeletal Radiol 1995;24(1):17–20.

Magnetic Resonance Imaging of the Glenoid Labrum

Michael B. Zlatkin, MD[a,b,*], Timothy G. Sanders, MD[a]

KEYWORDS

- Glenoid labrum • Shoulder • Instability • GIRD • ALPSA lesion • Bankart lesion • Perthes lesion
- GLAD lesion • SLAP lesion • Ganglion cyst

KEY POINTS

- The shoulder is inherently unstable and subject to injury.
- The labrum is one component of the shoulder mechanism that functions in preserving joint stability; it is also often a part of the pathologic lesions associated with instability, and isolated tears of the labrum associated with shoulder pain and dysfunction.
- Tears of the labrum are generally classified as anterior, posterior, inferior, and superior.
- The location and severity of the tear generally dictates clinical management, which may range from medical management to arthroscopic debridement and labral repair. In the more severe cases, a shoulder stabilization procedure may be needed.

INTRODUCTION

The shoulder is a joint capable of great freedom and motion. It is therefore both inherently unstable and subject to injury. Although the labrum is one component of the shoulder mechanism that functions in preserving joint stability, it is also often a part of the pathologic lesions associated with instability, and isolated tears of the labrum, such as superior labrum anterior posterior (SLAP) lesions, may also be associated with shoulder pain and dysfunction. The glenoid labrum is a redundant fold of the joint capsule made of fibrous and fibrocartilagenous tissue that attaches to the rim of the glenoid of the scapula. It deepens the glenoid fossa, provides an anchor for the long head of the biceps tendon, and provides an attachment for the remainder of the glenohumeral ligaments. Tears of the labrum are generally classified as anterior, posterior, inferior, and superior.

The location and severity of the tear generally dictates clinical management, which may range from medical management to arthroscopic debridement and labral repair. In the more severe cases, a shoulder stabilization procedure may be needed.

LABRAL ANATOMY

The glenoid labrum rims the glenoid cavity, and provides inherent stability to the glenohumeral joint, restricting anterior and posterior excursion of the humerus.[1] The labrum consists of hyaline cartilage, fibrocartilage, and fibrous tissue, but is mainly made up of parallel collagen fibers and dense fibrous connective tissue. Fibrocartilage is present in the labrum only in a small transition zone, at the attachment to the osseous glenoid rim. The blood supply of the labrum is mainly to the outermost portion of the labrum. The inner portion is without vessels.

The glenoid labrum is variable in size and thickness. The labral outline is ovoid in configuration, following the outline of the underlying glenoid rim. It is most firmly attached posteriorly and inferiorly. In young patients, the labrum is closely

[a] National Musculoskeletal Imaging (NMSI), Deerfield Beach, FL 33441, USA; [b] School of Medicine, University of Miami, Miami, FL 33124, USA
* Corresponding author.
E-mail address: mzlatkin@nationalrad.com

Radiol Clin N Am 51 (2013) 279–297
http://dx.doi.org/10.1016/j.rcl.2012.11.003
0033-8389/13/$ – see front matter © 2013 Elsevier Inc. All rights reserved.

attached at its base to the glenoid. There may be an abrupt transition, or there may be a transition zone where the fibrous labrum blends with the glenoid hyaline cartilage. In later years, especially the superior portion of the labrum may rest free on the edge of the glenoid. This may arise as a result of pull by the superior glenohumeral ligament and biceps tendon and may be distinguished from a labral tear by its smooth borders. In young athletes, superior quadrant labral tears may result from traction by these same 2 structures in overhead throwing.[2]

The glenoid labrum, by encircling the glenoid, enhances both the depth and surface area of the glenoid cavity, consequently improving congruity of the 2 articular surfaces.[3] It increases the surface area of the glenoid by approximately one-third.[4] The glenoid is also deepened by the thin cartilaginous lining in the center of this structure. It functions to provide nutrition to the glenoid cavity and helps maintain joint lubrication. It also acts to protect the chondral surface from compression and sheer damage. The labrum is also important as a site for ligamentous attachment,[5] as well as the biceps and triceps tendons. It acts as a valve that maintains negative intraarticular pressure and stability. It is believed that the strong intertwining between the collagen fibers of the glenohumeral ligaments and the labrum is more resistant to injury than the glenolabral junction/union.

The labrum can be divided into 4 quadrants: superior, anterior, inferior, and posterior (Fig. 1). There can be further division into anterior superior and anterior inferior and posterior inferior and posterior superior. Most pathologic lesions occur in the anterior inferior (Bankart lesions and their variants) and superior portions of the labrum (SLAP lesions). Alternatively, the labrum can be divided into a clock face with the most common designation using 12 o'clock to represent superior and 3 o'clock to represent anterior.

There appears to be a strong pathophysiologic relationship between the locations of labral lesions and the attachment sites of the glenohumeral ligaments and proximal biceps tendon.[6,7] The inferior portion of the labral-ligamentous complex is more important than the superior portion in stabilizing the glenohumeral joint. It is this portion of the labrum that is more commonly injured in patients with anterior glenohumeral instability. Nonetheless, the superior labrum does play some role in the stability of the glenohumeral joint, where it functions in conjunction with the biceps tendon, through the biceps labral complex. The superior and anterior superior portions of the labrum are the more variable in their attachment to the

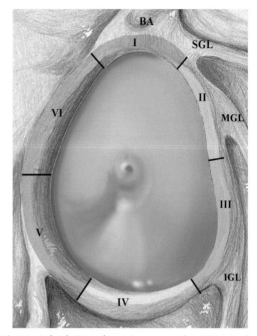

Fig. 1. Labral "quadrants": I, superior; II, anterior superior; III, anterior inferior; IV, inferior; V, posterior inferior; and VI, posterior superior. BA, biceps anchor; SGL, superior glenohumeral ligament; MGL, middle glenohumeral ligament; IGL, inferior glenohumeral ligament.

glenoid, whereas the more inferior portion of the labrum is typically fixed.

Initially, the labrum was considered to normally be of low signal intensity on all magnetic resonance (MR) pulse sequences; however, more recent studies have identified areas of increased linear or globular signal intensity in nearly a third of arthroscopically normal labral tissue.[8] Increased signal intensity in the labrum may also be caused by magic angle phenomenon,[9,10] particularly in the posterior superior aspect. Intermediate signal intensity may be noted at the chondrolabral junction corresponding to the transitional zone of fibrocartilage, which should not be misinterpreted as a labral tear.[11] Typically considered to be triangular or rounded in cross section, a range of glenoid labral morphologies has been described.[12] A triangular shape (Fig. 2) is most common (anterior, 64%; posterior, 47%), followed by rounded (17%, 33%). Flat, cleaved, notched, or absent labrum was also seen. The superior and anterior superior labrum may have a meniscoid shape. The labrum typically measures approximately 4 mm in width and 3 mm in thickness; however, broad variation in labral size from 2 to 14 mm among individuals exists, thus rendering size criteria of little diagnostic utility.[8]

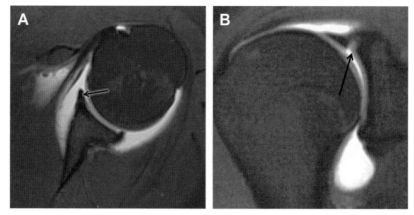

Fig. 2. Normal labrum, axial (*A*) and coronal (*B*) MR arthrographic images of the shoulder demonstrate a normal-appearing labrum (*short arrow*). The articular (hyaline) cartilage is intermediate in signal intensity. Articular cartilage undermining (*long arrow*) is noted as a normal anatomic variant in the superior quadrant.

The anterosuperior labrum, as well as the superior labrum, are common sites of normal anatomic variations, with specific variations described in up to 13.5% of those studied.[13–15] These variations in labral attachment occur above the equator of the glenoid, which occurs at the 3 o'clock position on the glenoid margin. Below the equator, the labrum should be firmly attached. The anterosuperior labrum is not attached to the bony glenoid in 8% to 12% of the population, referred to as a sublabral foramen, also known as a sublabral hole (**Fig. 3**).[16] This finding is located anterior to the biceps-labral complex.[17] A sublabral recess, also referred to as a sublabral sulcus, is a recess/synovial reflection between the biceps-labral complex and the superior margin of the glenoid (see **Fig. 3**).[16] On occasion, a sublabral recess can be continuous with a sublabral foramen.[17] In cadaver studies, a sublabral recess has been demonstrated in up to 73% of shoulders.[18] The anterosuperior labrum can also be focally absent, usually associated with a thickened, cordlike, middle glenohumeral ligament (**Fig. 4**). This entity is referred to as the Buford complex, believed to be present in approximately 1.5% of patients.[17] Pathologic lesions occurring or originating in, or extending

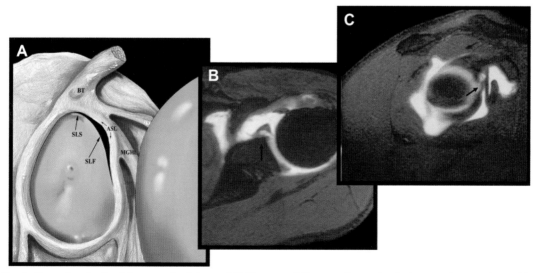

Fig. 3. Normal variants of the superior labrum. (*A*) Diagram of the superior and anterior superior quadrants. The sublabral sulcus or recess (SLS) is seen (*short arrow*). It may be continuous with the sublabral foramen, which is more anterior superior in location (SLF) (*long arrow*). BT, biceps tendon; ASL, anterior superior labrum; MGHL, middle glenohumeral ligament. Axial and sagittal MR arthrographic image of the shoulder (*B, C*) demonstrates the sublabral foramen (*arrow*).

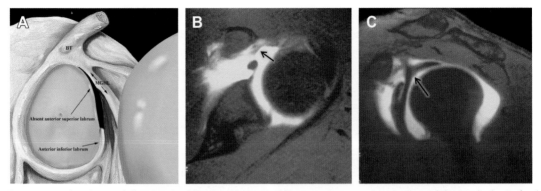

Fig. 4. Normal variants of the superior labrum. Diagram of the anterior superior quadrant (*A*) reveals the Buford complex. Note the absent anterior superior labrum (*long arrow*), and the thickened cordlike middle glenohumeral ligament (MGHL). Axial (*B*) and sagittal (*C*) MR arthrographic images of the shoulder demonstrate the absent anterosuperior labrum and thick cordlike MGHL (*arrows*).

into, the anterosuperior labral quadrant can also be distinguished from normal anatomic variations if they extend below the level of the coracoid process tip (which helps mark the equator) toward or into the anteroinferior labrum, or posteriorly into the posterosuperior quadrant (beyond the biceps labral anchor).[19] Therefore, a Buford complex should be suspected if the contiguous anteroinferior and superior labrum appear normal.[20] Morphologic alterations help to distinguish pathologic lesions as well. Other distinguishing features of SLAP lesions include extension laterally, irregular borders, and width on transverse MR images greater than 2 mm on MR imaging and 2.5 mm on MR arthrography.[21,22] MR arthrography may often delineate this anatomy to better advantage and help distinguish variant anatomy from pathologic lesions. These labral variants may, however, occur concomitantly with labral pathology, including SLAP lesions, and some studies have shown an increased incidence of such lesions in association with the aforementioned normal variants.[23–25] It is important to recognize these anatomic variations, as an unwitting repair of these structures may lead to diminished mobility.

Labral Lesions Associated with Shoulder Instability

General features

The shoulder is considered the most unstable joint in the human body. A simple definition of instability indicates that the humeral head slips out of its socket during activities. In the past, it was considered to be present only if a previous dislocation had occurred. Now more subtle degrees of instability are well recognized, including subluxation and instability that results from microtrauma.[26,27] Although the humeral head may translate a small amount during daily activities, in these more subtle types of instability, movement that then causes pain resulting from spasm or capsular stretching is what is then considered instability. The traditional forms of instability should be differentiated from glenohumeral joint laxity, in which asymptomatic passive translation of the humeral head on the glenoid fossa is observed. Glenohumeral joint laxity and instability may, however, coexist.

Instability may be classified according to frequency (acute, recurrent, or chronic), degree (subluxation or dislocation), etiology, and direction.[28,29] With regard to etiology, instability may result from one specific traumatic episode, and is called traumatic instability. It may also occur from repetitive microtrauma in activities, such as swimming or throwing. In addition, it may occur without any history of trauma and is termed atraumatic instability. These patients often have a coexistent history of congenital ligamentous laxity. Shoulder instability can also be described by direction, as anterior, posterior, or inferior to the glenoid, or multidirectional.[28,29] Anterior instability is by far the most common type of instability. Functional instability is another term that has also been used in the description of instability and it indicates that derangement of the shoulder is caused by damage that may be confined to the glenoid labrum.[30,31] The shoulder may catch, slip, or lock and may not exhibit subluxation or dislocation. Another term that is in current use to define different types of minor instability is microinstability. This is said to occur in some 5% of patients. It is a spectrum of disorders involving the upper one-half of the shoulder joint, as opposed to more traditional instability, which involves the lower one-third to one-half of the joint. Involved in the etiology of this process are such entities as a lax rotator interval, and there may also be history of overuse involved in these patients.[32,33]

Anterior Instability

Clinical features

Recurrent subluxation or dislocation (shoulder instability) is the most frequent complication of acute traumatic dislocation. When the initial event occurs between the ages of 15 and 35, the dislocations usually become recurrent or habitual.

True Bankart lesions are more commonly found in patients with a history of complete traumatic dislocation. In patients with a history of a subluxating shoulder, there may just be laxity or redundancy of the capsule, although labral lesions may also be seen.[34–38]

The "cartilaginous" lesion, as originally described by Bankart, has been considered to be an avulsion or tear of the glenoid labrum and/or stripping of the joint capsule. The damage to the anterior labrum that is seen at surgery, however, may vary from detachment of the labrum from the glenoid rim and tears of the substance of the labrum, to a completely destroyed or absent labrum.[30]

The labrum tears as it is avulsed by the glenohumeral ligaments at the time of injury. Failure of this complex at the glenoid side include the Bankart lesion described previously, but also includes its less common variants: the Perthes lesion and the anterior labroligamentous periosteal sleeve avulsion (ALPSA) lesion.

A typical Bankart lesion (fibrous Bankart lesion would be an avulsion of the labroligamentous complex from the anteroinferior portion of the glenoid.[39–41] The periosteum of the scapula is lifted and disrupted. It typically occurs at the 3-o'clock to 6-o'clock position, but may extend upward. The soft tissue lesion may be avulsed along with a piece of bone, the "bony" Bankart lesion, along the anteroinferior aspect of the glenoid rim.[42]

The axial imaging plane is the primary plane for detecting a Bankart lesion and MR imaging may demonstrate an irregular fluid or contrast collection extending into the substance of or deep to the labrum with or without abnormal morphology of the labrum.[43,44] As the adjacent medial scapular periosteum is often stripped from the adjacent bone or possibly completely disrupted, a displaced labral fragment (**Fig. 5**) may result. The location and extent of a labral tear should be described using either the quadrants of the glenoid as reference points or using the numbers of the face of the clock as reference points, as discussed in the anatomy section. The coronal imaging plane may also demonstrate fluid or contrast extending into the substance of the anterior inferior labrum, which has been described as the *double axillary pouch sign* (**Fig. 6**).

Bankart lesion variants

The previous discussion focuses on the typical lesion of anterior instability, the Bankart lesion, indicating an avulsion of the anterior inferior labrum, capsule, and inferior glenohumeral ligament complex, with an associated disruption of the scapular periosteum (see **Fig. 6**).[45–47] There are, however, a number of variants of this typical lesion.

Perthes Lesion

The Perthes lesion[48] is a nondisplaced tear of the anterior inferior glenoid labrum. It is a labral ligamentous avulsion in which the scapular periosteum remains intact but is stripped medially. The

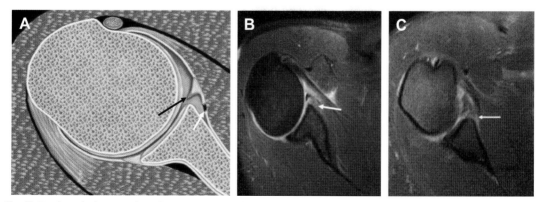

Fig. 5. Bankart lesion, MR imaging. Diagram in the axial plane reveals a tear and detachment of the anterior labrum (*black arrow*), with corresponding tear of the scapular periosteum (*white arrow*). Axial indirect MR arthrogram images (*A, B*) reveal a tear and detachment (*white arrow*) of the anterior inferior labrum. Also note some associated bone loss along the subjacent bony glenoid, but no bone Bankart fragment.

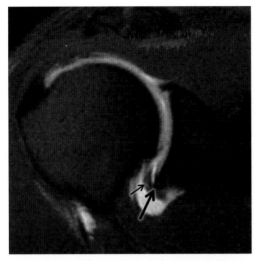

Fig. 6. Double axillary pouch sign, anterior labral tear in the coronal imaging plane. Coronal MR arthrographic image shows the double axillary pouch sign, a contrast collection (*long arrow*) located between the glenoid rim and torn anterior labrum (*short arrow*).

periosteum may then become redundant, and recurrent instability may occur as the humeral head moves forward into this region of acquired laxity (pseudojoint). The labrum may then lay back down into a relatively normal position on the glenoid, and resynovialize (heal back). It may then be very difficult to diagnose, as the detachment may not be easily identified on conventional MR imaging or even on MR arthrography (**Fig. 7**) (or at arthroscopy), unless specialized imaging positions, such as abducted and externally rotated (ABER), are used (see **Fig. 7**).[48–50] With distension from MR arthrography, and when needed with ABER positioning, only subtle displacement of the labral tissue may be seen.

ALPSA Lesion

In the ALPSA lesion (**Fig. 8**)[51,52] (medialized Bankart lesion), the scapular periosteum does not rupture, resulting in a medial displacement and inferior rotation of labroligamentous structures as they are stripped down to the scapular neck. The ALPSA lesion may then heal in this displaced position. A small cleft or separation can then be seen between the glenoid margin and the labrum. With a chronic ALPSA lesion, fibrous tissue is deposited on the medially displaced labral ligamentous complex, and the entire lesion then resynovializes along the articular surface. These lesions are easily detected in the acute setting, but may be more difficult to detect in the chronic setting when the medialized labral fragment has scarred down to the adjacent glenoid. This may leave a deformed and redundant labrum. This lesion may require more modified surgery than the typical Bankart lesion and therefore is important to recognize.[52–54] The lesion may require additional surgical debridement of the fibrosis and scar tissue before completing the Bankart repair. It is important to recognize before surgery as well, so that the labrum is not repaired in this medial location, thus losing the important bumper effect of the labrum at the margin of the glenoid. This is one of the more important causes of failed Bankart surgical repairs. In the absence of an effusion, the ALPSA lesion may be missed on conventional MR imaging if the lesion does not extend to the mid anterior labrum, as the fibrous medialized resynovialized mass may not be well seen on MR imaging in a patient with a paucity of joint fluid and magic angle artifact.[49] MR arthrography, including in the ABER position, may be valuable in revealing these lesions.

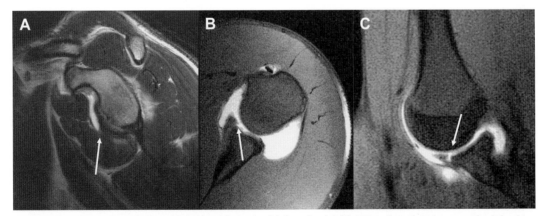

Fig. 7. Perthes lesion (nondisplaced labral tear). Sagittal (*A*) and axial (*B*) MR arthrogram images. The labral tear is difficult to discern, especially on the axial views. Axial oblique ABER MR arthrographic images demonstrate a collection of contrast (*long arrow*) extending partially beneath the anterior inferior labrum. The medial scapular periosteum remains intact, holding the labrum in near anatomic position.

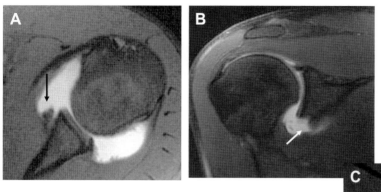

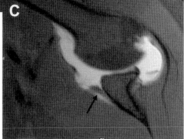

Fig. 8. ALPSA lesion (anterior labroligamentous periosteal sleeve avulsion), medialized Bankart. Axial (*A, B*) and ABER (*C*) MR arthrographic images demonstrate the torn anterior inferior labrum pulled in a medial direction (*arrows*) by an intact medial scapular periosteum.

The diagnostic performance of MR imaging and MR arthrography in the evaluation of labral tears has been evaluated. One study[55] of conventional MR imaging found a sensitivity of 93%, and a specificity 87%. Another larger study[43] found a sensitivity of 89%, and a specificity of 97%. MR imaging was found to be most sensitive in the evaluation of anterior labral tears, and less sensitive in superior and posterior tears. MR arthrography reveals a diagnostic performance similar to or better than conventional MR imaging and better reveals labral separation/detachment.[5,56–61]

Posterior Instability

Posterior instability of the shoulder is not as well understood, in part because it is uncommon but also because of the confusion in terminology differentiating posterior subluxations and dislocations.[28,45,46,62]

Isolated posterior instability is uncommon and accounts for only 5% of instability. Acute posterior dislocations of the glenohumeral joint are rare. They represent approximately 2% to 4% of all dislocations of the shoulder.[47,63] They may occur following trauma but are commonly associated with electric shock or seizures. Recurrence is not common.

Recurrence is common with atraumatic posterior dislocations and in patients with a history of a traumatic dislocation when large bony defects of the humerus and glenoid occur. Recurrent

posterior subluxation rather than dislocation is, however, the more common lesion. Overuse, as in athletics, is usually involved. Abduction, flexion, and internal rotation are the mechanisms involved (swimming, throwing, and punching), reflective of repeated microtrauma. These patients, often young athletes, may present with pain rather than signs of instability. There may be some association with posterior laxity.[45,46,62,64–70]

The posterior band of the inferior glenohumeral ligament is a primary static stabilizer of the glenohumeral joint with respect to translation posteriorly of the humeral head. Injury sufficient to cause posterior instability, however, requires injury to the posterior inferior labroligamentous complex as well as the posterior capsule. Labroligamentous findings in patients with prior posterior dislocations and resultant instability may be the reverse of those for recurrent anterior dislocations and include posterior labral and capsular detachments and tears, as well as posterior capsular laxity.[71] A reverse Bankart lesion consists of a tear of the posterior glenoid labrum (**Fig. 9**). The tear is often nondisplaced and seen on MR imaging as high-signal fluid or contrast extending into the substance or deep to the posterior labrum. A labral fragment may also be detached or displaced (see **Fig. 14**B). Posterior labrocapsular periosteal sleeve avulsion has also been described.[72,73]

Isolated lesions of the posterior labrum can occur after a single episode of trauma but may

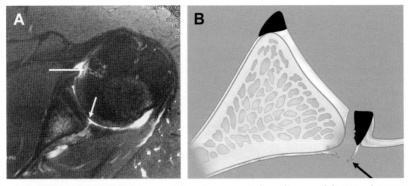

Fig. 9. Posterior instability. Axial T2 FS MRI image (*A*) and corresponding diagram (*B*). Note the torn and detached posterior labrum with disruption of the scapular periosteum posteriorly consistent with a reverse Bankart lesion (*white arrow* in *A*, *black arrow* in *B*). Note the reverse Hill Sachs lesion anteromedially in *A* (*longer white arrow*).

be more commonly related to multiple episodes and be microtraumatic in character (**Fig. 10**).[74,75] A 15-fold increase in posterior labral lesions has been documented in college football players. Although the etiology of the posterior labral tears is not definitely known, it may be caused by repetitive blocking during the sport or by weightlifting in these athletes, because the humeral head is repetitively jammed posteriorly into the posterior labrum during these activities.[75]

The MR and MR arthrographic findings associated with patients with posterior instability mirror those described for anterior instability, except they involve the posterior capsule and labrum.[67,76,77] MR imaging and MR arthrography may be used to identify the presence and extent of a tear and detachment of the posterior labroligamentous complex (see **Fig. 9**). Although the posterior capsule is injured, the capsular abnormalities may be less prominent than in anterior instability.[75,76]

Glenoid labrum articular disruption

Another recently described lesion occurs in athletes and has been described at arthroscopy.[78] This refers to tears of the superficial anterior inferior labrum and also involves the articular cartilage (see **Fig. 10**). This is the GLAD lesion (glenoid labrum articular disruption). This occurs from a forced adduction across the chest from an abducted and externally rotated position. There is impaction of the humeral head against the face of the glenoid. The labral tear is an inferior flap-type tear. There may be no history of dislocation or prominent findings of instability on physical examination. In addition, there is fibrillation and erosion of the articular cartilage in the anteroinferior quadrant of the glenoid fossa. These lesions may be visible on MR imaging (**Fig. 11**). MR arthrography may improve the sensitivity to these lesions.[79,80] Surgical treatment includes labral repair or debridement coupled with debridement of the chondral lesion.

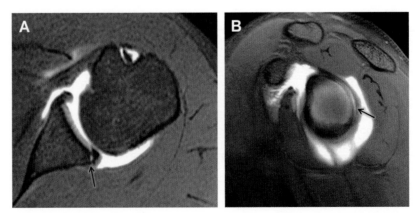

Fig. 10. Isolated posterior labral tear. Axial (*A*) and sagittal oblique (*B*) MR arthrogram images. Note the torn posterior labrum (*arrows*).

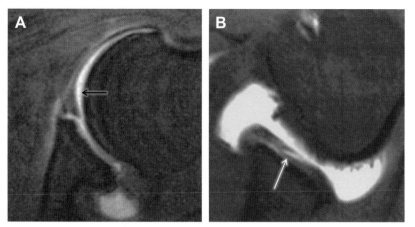

Fig. 11. GLAD lesion. Axial MR arthrogram images (*A*, *B*) demonstrate a nondisplaced tear of the anterior-inferior glenoid labrum (*black arrow*) with an adjacent chondral defect involving the anterior-inferior margin of the glenoid (*white arrow*).

Multiple labral lesions

The term "triple labral lesion" has been used to describe combined labral lesions involving the anterior, posterior, and superior labrum (Bankart, reverse-Bankart, and SLAP II) (**Fig. 12**). This should be differentiated from the term "triple lesion," which has been used to describe the progression of anterior-inferior labroligamentous damage with subsequent recurrent dislocations.[81] The triple labral lesion is not common according to the literature, seen in only 7 (2.4%) of 297 patients with labral tears in one study,[82] but some combination of labral lesions is not that uncommon in clinical practice. Most are thought to be the sequelae of primary anterior instability. This is supported by the "circle" concept of instability, which suggests that anterior instability requires a posterior capsular or labral injury in addition to a Bankart lesion for significant translation to occur. Posterior injury occurs as a "contrecoup lesion" and does not indicate posterior instability. Superior labral lesions may result in increased translation superior to inferior, and to a less prominent degree, anterior to posterior.

Combined lesions involving fewer than all 3 of the aforementioned portions of the labrum may also occur. Combined lesions of the anterior inferior labrum extending superiorly to involve the biceps anchor (superior labrum) are relatively common (SLAP V). Combined Bankart and reverse-Bankart lesions are seen less commonly than SLAP V lesions (**Fig. 13**). Combined reverse-Bankart and SLAP lesions may also be seen.

Arthroscopic treatment of triple labral lesions with suture anchors has been reported with good outcomes in 6 of 7 patients.[82] It is felt that repair of all 3 lesions is necessary to restore the circle of stability to the glenohumeral joint.

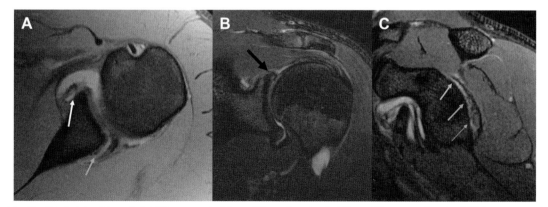

Fig. 12. Triple labral tear. Axial (*A*), coronal oblique (*B*), and sagittal oblique (*C*) proton-density (PD) fat-saturated images. Note the tear of the anterior (*white arrow* in *A*), superior (*black arrow* in *B*), and posterior (*shorter arrow* in *A*, *arrows* in *C*) labrum. The posterior labral tear is associated with a bone fragment.

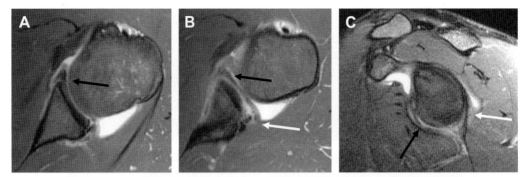

Fig. 13. Tear of the inferior labrum anterior and posterior. Indirect MR arthrogram images axial (A, B) and sagittal oblique (C). The labral tear extends anteroinferiorly (*black arrow*), posteroinferiorly (*white arrow*), and inferiorly.

SLAP lesions

Snyder and colleagues[83–85] introduced the term for defining injuries to the superior portion of the labrum and adjacent biceps tendon. A superior quadrant labral tear with anterior and posterior components of the tear is labeled an SLAP lesion. These lesions may be acute or chronic, and when acute, they may result from a fall on the outstretched arm, with the shoulder in abduction and forward flexion. It also may occur in athletes requiring repetitive overuse of the arm,[32,86–88] including baseball, tennis, or volleyball. The injury to the superior portion of the glenoid labrum may result from sudden forced abduction of the arm. It results from excessive traction related to sudden pull from the long head of the biceps tendon. The lesion may typically begin posteriorly and then extends anteriorly and terminates at or before the midglenoid notch. It includes the biceps labral anchor. In the throwing athlete, the late-cocking phase may be the most vulnerable time for labral injury. Labral variants may also predispose to SLAP lesions. SLAP tears were categorized into 4 basic types by Snyder and colleagues.[85] Type 1 reveals superior labral roughening and degeneration. The labrum remains firmly attached to the glenoid. These represent 10% of SLAP lesions. This lesion may represent a degenerative tear of the labrum. Type 2 is the most common lesion, and represents 40% of all SLAP lesions. Type 2 represents a detachment of this roughened superior portion of the labrum and its biceps tendon anchor (Fig. 14). Burkhart and colleagues[32,87] describe 3 distinct categories of type 2 SLAP lesions: (1) anterior, (2) posterior, and (3) combined anteroposterior. These investigators noted that type IIB (Fig. 15) and IIC lesions were more frequently observed than SLAP IIA lesions in throwing athletes.

Type 3 represents 30% of SLAP lesions. It is a bucket-handle tear of the superior portion of the labrum (Fig. 16). It does not involve the biceps labral anchor. At least half of the time, SLAP III lesions show the characteristic Cheerio sign, which is a rounded core of soft tissue surrounded by a rim of contrast material.[89] Type 4 represents 15% of SLAP lesions. It has, in addition to the bucket-handle tear, a split tear of the biceps tendon.

Maffet and colleagues[90] described 3 additional types of SLAP lesions after observing other patterns of biceps tendon superior labrum injury[57,86,91,92]: Type 5 is a Bankart lesion of the anterior inferior labrum that then extends superiorly to include separation of the biceps tendon anchor (Fig. 17). Type 6 lesions are unstable radial or flap tears that also involve separation of the biceps anchor. A type 7 lesion consists of anterior extension of the SLAP lesion to involve the middle glenohumeral ligament.

Nord and colleagues[90] described additional lesions, which include a type 8 lesion that extends posteroinferiorly (Fig. 18), with extensive detachment of the posterior labrum; a type 9 lesion, which is a complete concentric avulsion of the labrum circumferentially around the entire glenoid rim[88]; and a type 10 lesion, an SLAP lesion associated with a reverse-Bankart lesion.[90] Another type X lesion exists in the literature, which was described in 2000 as an SLAP lesion that extends into the rotator interval in the form of a lesion of the SGHL, coracohumeral ligament, capsule, or synovium.[93]

Snyder and colleagues'[85] classification remains the most popular. Others have studied the frequency of SLAP lesions, and Handelberg and colleagues[94] retrospectively reviewed 530 arthroscopies and discovered 32 SLAP lesions, 53% of which were type II. Kim and colleagues[86] prospectively reviewed 544 shoulder arthroscopy procedures and found 139 SLAP lesions, the most common being type I (74%) followed by type II

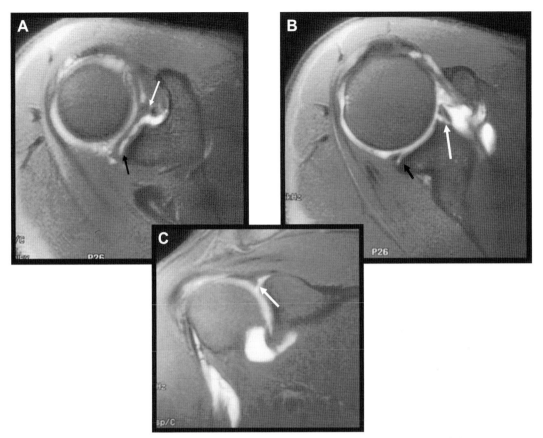

Fig. 14. SLAP 2 axial (*A, C*) and coronal oblique (*B*) MR arthrogram images, outlining a tear of the anterior superior (*white arrow in A, B*), posterior superior (*black arrow in A, white arrow in B*), and superior labrum (*white arrow in C*).

(21%), type IV (6%), and type III (0.7%). They discovered that although the most common type in their series was type I this was significantly associated with age. The topic of variability of diagnosis among experienced arthroscopists was studied by Gobezie and colleagues[95] (98 Ben) who, after viewing video vignettes of arthroscopies, found considerable intraobserver and interobserver variability among those deemed experts regarding both SLAP classification and

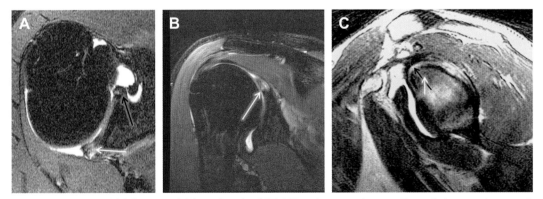

Fig. 15. SLAP 2 B. Axial (*A*), coronal (*B*), and sagittal (*C*) MR arthrogram images. Tear of the anterior superior (*black arrows*) and posterior superior labrum (*white arrows*) with posterior predominance, and some posterior inferior extension is best seen on the sagittal views.

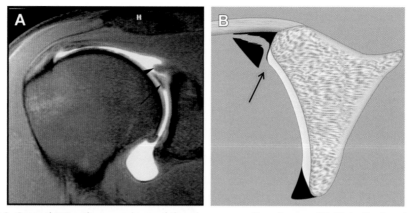

Fig. 16. SLAP 3. Coronal MR arthrogram image (*A*) and corresponding diagram (*B*). Note the tear in the superior labrum, with a separated fragment (*black arrow*) at the biceps labral anchor (*arrowhead*). Also note the partial tear along the undersurface of the supraspinatus tendon.

treatment. As arthroscopy is considered the gold standard on which many studies base their sensitivity, specificity, and predictive values, it is evident that, based on this study, reported values must be carefully scrutinized.

MR imaging and MR arthrography may be used in the detection of SLAP lesions.[57,89,91,96–100] In the study by Cartland and coworkers[101] on MR imaging examination, type 1 lesions exhibit irregularity of the labral contour with mildly increased signal intensity. Type 2 lesions may reveal a globular region of increased signal interposed between the superior labrum and glenoid margin. Type 3 shows typical linear increased signal extending to the labral surface. Type 4 lesions show high signal within the superior labrum, extending into the proximal biceps tendon. SLAP lesions may be difficult to detect on conventional MR imaging. The more superior portions of the tear can be difficult to visualize on axial images. External rotation, as well as coronal oblique images, help define these lesions.[89] MR arthrography can be very helpful in detecting SLAP lesions, including the use of traction in some select situations.[102] It will distend out buckle handle–type tears, outline morphologic alterations, and imbibe into areas of degeneration and fraying of the labrum and biceps tendon. MR arthrography demonstrates the following signs in SLAP lesions[103]: (1) contrast material may extend superiorly into the glenoid attachment of the long head of the biceps tendon (LHBT) on oblique coronal images, (2) irregularity of the insertion of the LHBT on oblique coronal and sagittal images, (3) accumulation of contrast material between the labrum and glenoid fossa on axial images, (4) detachment and displacement of the superior labrum on oblique sagittal and coronal images, or (5) a fragment of the labrum displaced inferiorly between the glenoid fossa and the humeral head. In addition, as noted in the following section, a paralabral cyst may be frequently associated with these lesions. Sensitivity, specificity, and accuracy of MR imaging have been reported to be between 66% and 98%, 71% and 90%, and 77% and 96%, respectively.[104,105] Sensitivity, specificity, and accuracy of direct MR arthrography has been reported to be between 82% and 100%, 69% and 98%, and 74% and 94%, respectively.[91,96,106] MR imaging has been less impressive in defining the particular

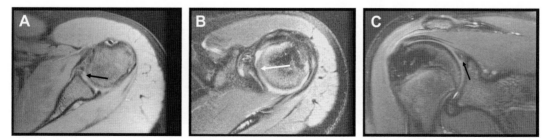

Fig. 17. SLAP 5. Axial (*A, B*), coronal oblique (*C*) PD fat-saturated images. Note the tear of the anterior (*black arrow* in *A*), anterior superior (*white arrow* in *B*), and posterior superior labrum (*black arrow* in *C*).

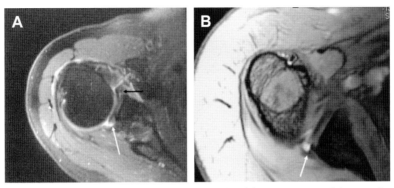

Fig. 18. SLAP 8. Axial PD fat-saturated (*A*) and T2* gradient-echo (*B*) images. Tear of the anterior superior (*black arrow*) and posterior superior (*white arrow* in *A*) labrum, with posterior inferior extension, (*white arrow* in *B*).

type of SLAP lesion, regardless of modality. Improved detection of SLAP lesions is possible with the arm in an ABER position,[107,108] and with the arm in traction. SLAP lesions are frequently associated with rotator cuff lesions, particularly partial tears. One study found such lesions in 42% of cases.[91]

PARALABRAL GANGLION CYSTS

These are ganglion cysts arising adjacent to the glenoid labrum[109–111] and most commonly associated with a labral tear (**Fig. 19**). This labral tear is often an SLAP lesion and the paralabral cyst most commonly arises in relation to the posterosuperior component. They may, however, occur anywhere in the glenohumeral joint. Pathophysiologically, they may be similar to cysts of this nature elsewhere in the body, such as meniscal cysts or cysts associated with tears of the acetabular labrum. In this situation, fluid arising from the joint extends through the labral tear into the surrounding soft tissues and leads to ganglion cyst formation. Paralabral cysts may be difficult to identify on MR

arthrography, unless some form of T2-weighted sequence is performed, as direct communication between a cyst and the joint space rarely occurs. A posterior or inferior cyst may cause compression neuropathy of the suprascapular or axillary nerve, respectively. Compression of the suprascapular nerve is usually with extension of the posterior cyst into the spinoglenoid notch. Nerve compression can result in denervation of the muscles enervated by the affected nerve. In the acute setting, the muscle will demonstrate diffuse edema; at this point, the muscle and nerve damage is still considered to be reversible. In the chronic setting, muscle edema is replaced by fatty atrophy/fatty infiltration of the involved muscle. At this point, the nerve and muscle damage is considered irreversible. Compression of the suprascapular nerve at the level of the suprascapular notch results in denervation of both the supraspinatus and infraspinatus muscles, whereas compression of the nerve at the level of the spinoglenoid notch results in isolated denervation of the infraspinatus muscle, as the branch to the supraspinatus muscle has already been given off. Compression of the axillary

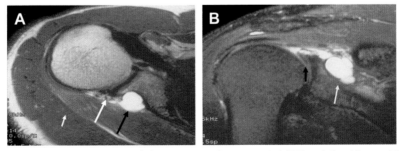

Fig. 19. Paralabral cyst with compression of the suprascapular nerve. Axial T2-weighted image (*A*) demonstrates a tear (*white arrow*) of the posterior superior abrum with an associated paralabral cyst (*black arrow*) dissecting into the spinoglenoid notch posteriorly. Coronal PD fat-saturated image (*B*) shows the paralabral cyst (*white arrow*) dissecting into the spinoglenoid notch posteriorly. There is early atrophy (*short white arrow* in *A*) isolated to the infraspinatus muscle, indicating chronic compression of the suprascapular nerve at the level of the spinoglenoid notch.

nerve generally results in denervation of the teres minor and sometimes the deltoid muscle.[112] Cysts that cause nerve compression are usually large (mean size 3.1 cm).

LABRAL LESIONS ASSOCIATED WITH THROWING

Current understanding of the biomechanics of throwing suggests that most injuries occur either during the *late-cocking phase* with the arm positioned in maximum abduction and external rotation or as a result of the tremendous forces that are generated across the glenohumeral joint during the *acceleration* and *deceleration* phases of throwing.[32,113] The term "dead arm" has been coined to describe a pathologic condition in which a throwing athlete is unable to continue to throw with the same accuracy or control as a result of pain or as a result of a subjective unease in the shoulder.

Jobe[114] put forth the theory of *internal impingement* to explain the dead arm syndrome in certain throwing athletes. With *intrinsic impingement,* the primary cause of the lesion is again thought to be anterior capsular stretching resulting from repetitive microtrauma to these structures during the late-cocking and early-acceleration phases of throwing. In internal impingement, the lesions occur as a result of the impingement of the undersurface of the posterior cuff between the posterior aspect of the greater tuberosity and the posterosuperior labrum.[114] This theory of internal impingement put forth by Jobe and Walsh supports the idea of anterior capsular stretching as the primary lesion in throwing athletes. The lesions of internal impingement are seen as tendinosis and partial thickness articular sided tears of the posterior cuff combined with posterior superior labral tears.

MR imaging typically demonstrates some combination of 4 abnormalities (**Fig. 20**). These include (1) tendinosis and/or partial thickness–articular-sided tearing of the posterior cuff, (2) abnormal signal or a frank tear of the posterosuperior labrum, (3) marrow edema and/or subcortical cystic change within the posterior aspect of the humeral head, and (4) internal impingement seen on ABER imaging. The presence of abnormalities of the posterior cuff combined with an abnormality of the superior labrum in the symptomatic overhead athlete appears to be most sensitive with regard to the diagnosis of internal impingement.[115,116] These lesions of the posterior cuff and superior labrum can be quite subtle and the use of direct MR arthrography can improve

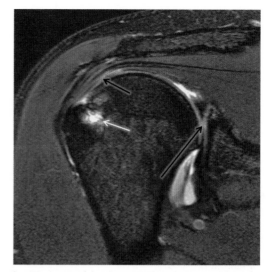

Fig. 20. Internal impingement. A 24-year-old professional baseball pitcher demonstrates changes of internal impingement. Coronal MR arthrographic image demonstrates fraying, irregularity, and a tear of the posterior superior labrum (*long black arrow*), tendinosis and partial-thickness articular-sided tear of the infraspinatus tendon (*shorter black arrow*), and subcortical cystic change and marrow edema of the greater tuberosity (*white arrow*).

detection of these lesions in the young overhead athlete with symptoms of internal impingement.

Glenohumeral Internal Rotation Deficit Disorder

Glenohumeral internal rotation deficit disorder (GIRD), as put forth by Burkhart and colleagues,[32,113] suggests that the primary lesion in many overhead athletes is not a stretching of the anterior capsule, but rather scarring and fibrosis of the posterior capsule or tightening of the posterior cuff musculature secondary to repetitive overhead activity. This theory suggests that the primary lesion is one of posterior capsular tightness rather than anterior capsular laxity that leads to the various lesions of the labrum and rotator cuff in the "dead arm" syndrome. It is theorized that posterior capsular scarring or posterior muscle tightness pulls the humeral head in a posterior direction, shifting the humeral head "point of contact" on the face of the glenoid in a posterosuperior direction during the late-cocking phase of throwing. This results in a loss of internal rotation of the glenohumeral joint to less than 180° when compared with the non-throwing arm.

In GIRD, it is theorized that the posterior capsular scarring or posterior muscle tightening results from repetitive trauma to the posterior

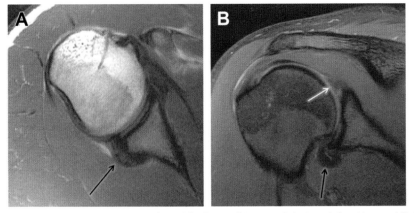

Fig. 21. An 18-year-old baseball pitcher with clinical findings of GIRD. Axial PD-weighted image (*A*) demonstrates marked thickening (*black arrow*) of the posterior capsule. Coronal PD fat-saturated image also shows signs of internal impingement with tendinosis of the infraspinatus tendon and signal alterations within the posterosuperior labrum (*white arrow* in *B*). The thickened posterior inferior capsule is again noted (*black arrow*).

shoulder during the late-cocking phase of throwing. This results in a cascade of injuries, beginning with a posterosuperior shift of the "point of contact" of the humeral head on the glenoid face during the late-cocking phase of throwing. Loss of internal rotation of the glenohumeral joint of the throwing arm ensues and, as a result, during the late-cocking phase of throwing, abnormal twisting rotational forces are applied to the anchor of the long of the biceps tendon and a *peel-back* injury occurs to the posterior superior labrum during the acceleration phase of throwing, resulting in a tear of the posterosuperior labrum. These changes of the posterior capsule and posterosuperior labrum are often seen in conjunction with changes of the posterior cuff resulting from internal impingement.

The MR findings associated with GIRD (**Fig. 21**) include a focal area of thickening or fibrosis of the posterior capsule immediately adjacent to the glenoid attachment. Also, the changes of internal impingement, including abnormalities of the posterior cuff and greater tuberosity, are seen. Finally, a peel-back or avulsion-type lesion of the posterior superior labrum may be seen.[117]

Preventive treatment for GIRD includes posterior capsule/muscle-stretching exercises after each pitching outing, which has been shown to decrease the incidence of GIRD in the highly competitive overhead athlete. Once a labral lesion occurs, treatment includes SLAP repair of the peel-back lesion, rather than debridement and rotator cuff debridement or repair as needed. Early results suggest a 70% to 80% return to pre-injury level of activity.[32,113,117]

REFERENCES

1. Carson WG Jr. Arthroscopy of the shoulder: anatomy and technique. Orthop Rev 1992;21: 143–53.
2. Andrews JR, Carson WG Jr, McLeod WD. Glenoid labrum tears related to the long head of the biceps. Am J Sports Med 1985;13:337–41.
3. Howell SM, Galinat BJ. The glenoid-labral socket. A constrained articular surface. Clin Orthop Relat Res 1989;243:122–5.
4. Moon YL, Singh H, Yang H, et al. Arthroscopic rotator interval closure by purse string suture for symptomatic inferior shoulder instability. Orthopedics 2011;34.
5. Beltran J, Rosenberg ZS, Chandnani VP, et al. Glenohumeral instability: evaluation with MR arthrography. Radiographics 1997;17:657–73.
6. Palmer WE. MR arthrography of the rotator cuff and labral-ligamentous complex. Semin Ultrasound CT MR 1997;18:278–90.
7. Palmer WE, Caslowitz PL, Chew FS. MR arthrography of the shoulder: normal intraarticular structures and common abnormalities. AJR Am J Roentgenol 1995;164:141–6.
8. Zanetti M, Carstensen T, Weishaupt D, et al. MR arthrographic variability of the arthroscopically normal glenoid labrum: qualitative and quantitative assessment. Eur Radiol 2001;11:559–66.
9. Tuoheti Y, Itoi E, Minagawa H, et al. Attachment types of the long head of the biceps tendon to the glenoid labrum and their relationships with the glenohumeral ligaments. Arthroscopy 2005;21: 1242–9.
10. Kolts I, Busch LC, Tomusk H, et al. Anatomical composition of the anterior shoulder joint capsule.

A cadaver study on 12 glenohumeral joints. Ann Anat 2001;183:53–9.

11. Loredo R, Longo C, Salonen D, et al. Glenoid labrum: MR imaging with histologic correlation. Radiology 1995;196:33–41.

12. Park YH, Lee JY, Moon SH, et al. MR arthrography of the labral capsular ligamentous complex in the shoulder: imaging variations and pitfalls. AJR Am J Roentgenol 2000;175:667–72.

13. Tuite MJ, Blankenbaker DG, Seifert M, et al. Sublabral foramen and Buford complex: inferior extent of the unattached or absent labrum in 50 patients. Radiology 2002;223:137–42.

14. Beltran J, Bencardino J, Mellado J, et al. MR arthrography of the shoulder: variants and pitfalls. Radiographics 1997;17:1403–12 [discussion: 1412–05].

15. Tuite MJ, Orwin JF. Anterosuperior labral variants of the shoulder: appearance on gradient-recalled-echo and fast spin-echo MR images. Radiology 1996;199:537–40.

16. Kwak SM, Brown RR, Resnick D, et al. Anatomy, anatomic variations, and pathology of the 11- to 3-o'clock position of the glenoid labrum: findings on MR arthrography and anatomic sections. AJR Am J Roentgenol 1998;171:235–8.

17. Stoller DW. MR arthrography of the glenohumeral joint. Radiol Clin North Am 1997;35:97–116.

18. Smith DK, Chopp TM, Aufdemorte TB, et al. Sublabral recess of the superior glenoid labrum: study of cadavers with conventional nonenhanced MR imaging, MR arthrography, anatomic dissection, and limited histologic examination. Radiology 1996;201:251–6.

19. Tsao LY, Mirowitz SA. MR imaging of the shoulder. Imaging techniques, diagnostic pitfalls, and normal variants. Magn Reson Imaging Clin N Am 1997;5:683–704.

20. Tirman PF, Feller JF, Palmer WE, et al. The Buford complex—a variation of normal shoulder anatomy: MR arthrographic imaging features. AJR Am J Roentgenol 1996;166:869–73.

21. Waldt S, Metz S, Burkart A, et al. Variants of the superior labrum and labro-bicipital complex: a comparative study of shoulder specimens using MR arthrography, multi-slice CT arthrography and anatomical dissection. Eur Radiol 2006;16:451–8.

22. Tuite MJ, Rutkowski A, Enright T, et al. Width of high signal and extension posterior to biceps tendon as signs of superior labrum anterior to posterior tears on MRI and MR arthrography. AJR Am J Roentgenol 2005;185:1422–8.

23. Ilahi OA, Cosculluela PE, Ho DM. Classification of anterosuperior glenoid labrum variants and their association with shoulder pathology. Orthopedics 2008;31:226.

24. Rao AG, Kim TK, Chronopoulos E, et al. Anatomical variants in the anterosuperior aspect of the glenoid labrum: a statistical analysis of seventy-three cases. J Bone Joint Surg Am 2003;85-A:653–9.

25. Bents RT, Skeete KD. The correlation of the Buford complex and SLAP lesions. J Shoulder Elbow Surg 2005;14:565–9.

26. Wall MS, O'Brien SJ. Arthroscopic evaluation of the unstable shoulder. Clin Sports Med 1995;14:817–39.

27. O'Brien SJ, Neves MC, Arnoczky SP, et al. The anatomy and histology of the inferior glenohumeral ligament complex of the shoulder. Am J Sports Med 1990;18:449–56.

28. Schwartz E, Warren RF, O'Brien SJ, et al. Posterior shoulder instability. Orthop Clin North Am 1987;18:409–19.

29. O'Brien SJ, Warren RF, Schwartz E. Anterior shoulder instability. Orthop Clin North Am 1987;18:395–408.

30. Zarins B, McMahon MS, Rowe CR. Diagnosis and treatment of traumatic anterior instability of the shoulder. Clin Orthop 1993;(291):75–84.

31. Zarins B, Rowe CR. Current concepts in the diagnosis and treatment of shoulder instability in athletes. Med Sci Sports Exerc 1984;16:444–8.

32. Burkhart SS, Morgan CD, Kibler WB. The disabled throwing shoulder: spectrum of pathology. Part I: pathoanatomy and biomechanics. Arthroscopy 2003;19:404–20.

33. Sperling JW, Anderson K, McCarty EC, et al. Complications of thermal capsulorrhaphy. Instr Course Lect 2001;50:37–41.

34. Werner CM, Jacob HA, Dumont CE, et al. Static anterior glenohumeral subluxation following coracoid bone block in combination with pectoralis major transfer: a case report and biomechanical considerations. Rev Chir Orthop Reparatrice Appar Mot 2004;90:156–60 [in French].

35. Postacchini F, Mancini A. Anterior instability of the shoulder due to capsular laxity. Ital J Orthop Traumatol 1988;14:175–85.

36. Rowe CR. Recurrent anterior transient subluxation of the shoulder. The "dead arm" syndrome. Orthop Clin North Am 1988;19:767–72.

37. Rowe CR, Zarins B. Recurrent transient subluxation of the shoulder. J Bone Joint Surg Am 1981;63:863–72.

38. Morton KS. The unstable shoulder: recurring subluxation. Injury 1979;10:304–6.

39. Massengill AD, Seeger LL, Yao L, et al. Labrocapsular ligamentous complex of the shoulder: normal anatomy, anatomic variation, and pitfalls of MR imaging and MR arthrography. Radiographics 1994;14:1211–23.

40. O'Neill DB. Arthroscopic Bankart repair of anterior detachments of the glenoid labrum. A prospective study. J Bone Joint Surg Am 1999;81:1357–66.

41. Cole BJ, L'Insalata J, Irrgang J, et al. Comparison of arthroscopic and open anterior shoulder stabilization. A two to six-year follow-up study. J Bone Joint Surg Am 2000;82:1108–14.

42. Edelson JG. Bony changes of the glenoid as a consequence of shoulder instability. J Shoulder Elbow Surg 1996;5:293–8.

43. Gusmer PB, Potter HG, Schatz JA, et al. Labral injuries: accuracy of detection with unenhanced MR imaging of the shoulder. Radiology 1996;200:519–24.

44. Palmer WE, Brown JH, Rosenthal DI. Labral-ligamentous complex of the shoulder: evaluation with MR arthrography. Radiology 1994;190:645–51.

45. Tibone JE, Bradley JP. The treatment of posterior subluxation in athletes. Clin Orthop 1993;(291):124–37.

46. Hawkins RJ, Belle RM. Posterior instability of the shoulder. Instr Course Lect 1989;38:211–5.

47. Pavlov H, Warren RF, Weiss CB Jr, et al. The roentgenographic evaluation of anterior shoulder instability. Clin Orthop 1985;(194):153–8.

48. Wischer TK, Bredella MA, Genant HK, et al. Perthes lesion (a variant of the Bankart lesion): MR imaging and MR arthrographic findings with surgical correlation. AJR Am J Roentgenol 2002;178:233–7.

49. Tirman PF, Palmer WE, Feller JF. MR arthrography of the shoulder. Magn Reson Imaging Clin N Am 1997;5:811–39.

50. Tirman PF, Bost FW, Steinbach LS, et al. MR arthrographic depiction of tears of the rotator cuff: benefit of abduction and external rotation of the arm. Radiology 1994;192:851–6.

51. Connell DA, Potter HG. Magnetic resonance evaluation of the labral capsular ligamentous complex: a pictorial review. Australas Radiol 1999;43:419–26.

52. Neviaser TJ. The anterior labroligamentous periosteal sleeve avulsion lesion: a cause of anterior instability of the shoulder. Arthroscopy 1993;9:17–21.

53. Sailer J, Imhof H. Shoulder instability. Radiologe 2004;44:578–90 [in German].

54. Yoneda M. Neviaser's contribution to the treatment of ALPSA lesions. J Bone Joint Surg Am 2001;83-A:621–2.

55. Iannotti JP, Zlatkin MB, Esterhai JL, et al. Magnetic resonance imaging of the shoulder. Sensitivity, specificity, and predictive value. J Bone Joint Surg Am 1991;73:17–29.

56. McCauley TR. MR imaging of the glenoid labrum. Magn Reson Imaging Clin N Am 2004;12:97–109, vi–vii.

57. Beltran J, Jbara M, Maimon R. Shoulder: labrum and bicipital tendon. Top Magn Reson Imaging 2003;14:35–49.

58. Tuite MJ, Rubin D. CT and MR arthrography of the glenoid labroligamentous complex. Semin Musculoskelet Radiol 1998;2:363–76.

59. Chandnani VP, Gagliardi JA, Murnane TG, et al. Glenohumeral ligaments and shoulder capsular mechanism: evaluation with MR arthrography. Radiology 1995;196:27–32.

60. Tirman PF, Stauffer AE, Crues JV 3rd, et al. Saline magnetic resonance arthrography in the evaluation of glenohumeral instability. Arthroscopy 1993;9:550–9.

61. Habibian A, Stauffer A, Resnick D, et al. Comparison of conventional and computed arthrotomography with MR imaging in the evaluation of the shoulder. J Comput Assist Tomogr 1989;13:968–75.

62. Hawkins RJ, Janda DH. Posterior instability of the glenohumeral joint. A technique of repair. Am J Sports Med 1996;24:275–8.

63. Pavlov H, Freiberger RH. Fractures and dislocations about the shoulder. Semin Roentgenol 1978;13:85–96.

64. Tuite MJ. MR imaging of sports injuries to the rotator cuff. Magn Reson Imaging Clin N Am 2003;11:207–19, v.

65. Abrams JS. Arthroscopic repair of posterior instability and reverse humeral glenohumeral ligament avulsion lesions. Orthop Clin North Am 2003;34:475–83.

66. Kim SH, Ha KI, Park JH, et al. Arthroscopic posterior labral repair and capsular shift for traumatic unidirectional recurrent posterior subluxation of the shoulder. J Bone Joint Surg Am 2003;85-A:1479–87.

67. Tung GA, Hou DD. MR arthrography of the posterior labrocapsular complex: relationship with glenohumeral joint alignment and clinical posterior instability. AJR Am J Roentgenol 2003;180:369–75.

68. Hovis WD, Dean MT, Mallon WJ, et al. Posterior instability of the shoulder with secondary impingement in elite golfers. Am J Sports Med 2002;30:886–90.

69. Misamore GW, Facibene WA. Posterior capsulorrhaphy for the treatment of traumatic recurrent posterior subluxations of the shoulder in athletes. J Shoulder Elbow Surg 2000;9:403–8.

70. Weinberg J, McFarland EG. Posterior capsular avulsion in a college football player. Am J Sports Med 1999;27:235–7.

71. Petersen SA. Posterior shoulder instability. Orthop Clin North Am 2000;31:263–74.

72. Yu JS, Ashman CJ, Jones G. The POLPSA lesion: MR imaging findings with arthroscopic correlation

in patients with posterior instability. Skeletal Radiol 2002;31:396–9.

73. Simons P, Joekes E, Nelissen RG, et al. Posterior labrocapsular periosteal sleeve avulsion complicating locked posterior shoulder dislocation. Skeletal Radiol 1998;27:588–90.

74. Escobedo EM, Richardson ML, Schulz YB, et al. Increased risk of posterior glenoid labrum tears in football players. AJR Am J Roentgenol 2007;188: 193–7.

75. Shah N, Tung GA. Imaging signs of posterior glenohumeral instability. AJR Am J Roentgenol 2009; 192:730–5.

76. Rafii M, Firooznia H, Golimbu C. MR imaging of glenohumeral instability. Magn Reson Imaging Clin N Am 1997;5:787–809.

77. Jerosch J, Castro WH, Assheuer J. Nuclear magnetic resonance tomography diagnosis of changes in the glenoid process in patients with unstable shoulder joints. Sportverletz Sportschaden 1992;6:106–12 [in German].

78. Neviaser TJ. The GLAD lesion: another cause of anterior shoulder pain. Arthroscopy 1993;9:22–3.

79. Amrami KK, Sperling JW, Bartholmai BJ, et al. Radiologic case study. Glenolabral articular disruption (GLAD) lesion. Orthopedics 2002;25: 29, 95–6.

80. Sanders TG, Tirman PF, Linares R, et al. The glenolabral articular disruption lesion: MR arthrography with arthroscopic correlation. AJR Am J Roentgenol 1999;172:171–5.

81. Habermeyer P, Gleyze P, Rickert M. Evolution of lesions of the labrum-ligament complex in posttraumatic anterior shoulder instability: a prospective study. J Shoulder Elbow Surg 1999;8:66–74.

82. Lo IK, Burkhart SS. Triple labral lesions: pathology and surgical repair technique—report of seven cases. Arthroscopy 2005;21:186–93.

83. Snyder SJ, Banas MP, Belzer JP. Arthroscopic evaluation and treatment of injuries to the superior glenoid labrum. Instr Course Lect 1996;45: 65–70.

84. Snyder SJ, Banas MP, Karzel RP. An analysis of 140 injuries to the superior glenoid labrum. J Shoulder Elbow Surg 1995;4:243–8.

85. Snyder SJ, Karzel RP, Del Pizzo W, et al. SLAP lesions of the shoulder. Arthroscopy 1990;6:274–9.

86. Kim TK, Queale WS, Cosgarea AJ, et al. Clinical features of the different types of SLAP lesions: an analysis of one hundred and thirty-nine cases. J Bone Joint Surg Am 2003;85:66–71.

87. Burkhart SS, Morgan CD, Kibler WB. Shoulder injuries in overhead athletes. The "dead arm" revisited. Clin Sports Med 2000;19:125–58.

88. Mileski RA, Snyder SJ. Superior labral lesions in the shoulder: pathoanatomy and surgical management. J Am Acad Orthop Surg 1998;6:121–31.

89. Monu JU, Pope TL Jr, Chabon SJ, et al. MR diagnosis of superior labral anterior posterior (SLAP) injuries of the glenoid labrum: value of routine imaging without intraarticular injection of contrast material. AJR Am J Roentgenol 1994; 163:1425–9.

90. Nord KD, Brady PC, Yazdani RS, et al. The anatomy and function of the low posterolateral portal in addressing posterior labral pathology. Arthroscopy 2007;23:999–1005.

91. Bencardino JT, Beltran J, Rosenberg ZS, et al. Superior labrum anterior-posterior lesions: diagnosis with MR arthrography of the shoulder. Radiology 2000;214:267–71.

92. Maffet MW, Gartsman GM, Moseley B. Superior labrum-biceps tendon complex lesions of the shoulder. Am J Sports Med 1995;23:93–8.

93. Chang EY, Fliszar E, Chung CB. Superior labrum anterior and posterior lesions and microinstability. Magn Reson Imaging Clin N Am 2012;20:277–94, x–xi.

94. Handelberg F, Willems S, Shahabpour M, et al. SLAP lesions: a retrospective multicenter study. Arthroscopy 1998;14:856–62.

95. Gobezie R, Zurakowski D, Lavery K, et al. Analysis of interobserver and intraobserver variability in the diagnosis and treatment of SLAP tears using the Snyder classification. Am J Sports Med 2008;36: 1373–9.

96. Waldt S, Burkart A, Lange P, et al. Diagnostic performance of MR arthrography in the assessment of superior labral anteroposterior lesions of the shoulder. AJR Am J Roentgenol 2004;182: 1271–8.

97. Jee WH, McCauley TR, Katz LD, et al. Superior labral anterior posterior (SLAP) lesions of the glenoid labrum: reliability and accuracy of MR arthrography for diagnosis. Radiology 2001;218:127–32.

98. De Maeseneer M, Van Roy F, Lenchik L, et al. CT and MR arthrography of the normal and pathologic anterosuperior labrum and labral-bicipital complex. Radiographics 2000;20(Spec No):S67–81.

99. Tung GA, Entzian D, Green A, et al. High-field and low-field MR imaging of superior glenoid labral tears and associated tendon injuries. AJR Am J Roentgenol 2000;174:1107–14.

100. Smith AM, McCauley TR, Jokl P. SLAP lesions of the glenoid labrum diagnosed with MR imaging. Skeletal Radiol 1993;22:507–10.

101. Cartland JP, Crues JV 3rd, Stauffer A, et al. MR imaging in the evaluation of SLAP injuries of the shoulder: findings in 10 patients. AJR Am J Roentgenol 1992;159:787–92.

102. Chan KK, Muldoon KA, Yeh L, et al. Superior labral anteroposterior lesions: MR arthrography with arm traction. AJR Am J Roentgenol 1999;173: 1117–22.

103. Shankman S, Bencardino J, Beltran J. Glenohumeral instability: evaluation using MR arthrography of the shoulder. Skeletal Radiol 1999;28:365–82.

104. Connell DA, Potter HG, Wickiewicz TL, et al. Noncontrast magnetic resonance imaging of superior labral lesions: 102 cases confirmed at arthroscopic surgery. Am J Sports Med 1999;27:208–13.

105. Dinauer PA, Flemming DJ, Murphy KP, et al. Diagnosis of superior labral lesions: comparison of noncontrast MRI with indirect MR arthrography in unexercised shoulders. Skeletal Radiol 2007;36: 195–202.

106. Applegate GR, Hewitt M, Snyder SJ, et al. Chronic labral tears: value of magnetic resonance arthrography in evaluating the glenoid labrum and labral-bicipital complex. Arthroscopy 2004;20:959–63.

107. Choi JA, Suh SI, Kim BH, et al. Comparison between conventional MR arthrography and abduction and external rotation MR arthrography in revealing tears of the antero-inferior glenoid labrum. Korean J Radiol 2001;2:216–21.

108. Cvitanic O, Tirman PF, Feller JF, et al. Using abduction and external rotation of the shoulder to increase the sensitivity of MR arthrography in revealing tears of the anterior glenoid labrum. AJR Am J Roentgenol 1997;169:837–44.

109. Sherman PM, Sanders TG, De Lone DR. A benign soft tissue mass simulating a glenoid labral cyst on unenhanced magnetic resonance imaging. Mil Med 2004;169:376–8.

110. Mellado JM, Salvado E, Camins A, et al. Fluid collections and juxta-articular cystic lesions of the shoulder: spectrum of MRI findings. Eur Radiol 2002;12:650–9.

111. Tung GA, Entzian D, Stern JB, et al. MR imaging and MR arthrography of paraglenoid labral cysts. AJR Am J Roentgenol 2000;174:1707–15.

112. Sanders TG, Tirman PF. Paralabral cyst: an unusual cause of quadrilateral space syndrome. Arthroscopy 1999;15:632–7.

113. Burkhart SS, Morgan CD, Kibler WB. The disabled throwing shoulder: spectrum of pathology. Part II: evaluation and treatment of SLAP lesions in throwers. Arthroscopy 2003;19:531–9.

114. Jobe CM. Superior glenoid impingement. Orthop Clin North Am 1997;28:137–43.

115. Giaroli EL, Major NM, Higgins LD. MRI of internal impingement of the shoulder. AJR Am J Roentgenol 2005;185:925–9.

116. Grainger AJ. Internal impingement syndromes of the shoulder. Semin Musculoskelet Radiol 2008; 12:127–35.

117. Tuite MJ, Petersen BD, Wise SM, et al. Shoulder MR arthrography of the posterior labrocapsular complex in overhead throwers with pathologic internal impingement and internal rotation deficit. Skeletal Radiol 2007;36:495–502.

Wrist Injuries
A Comparison Between High- and Low-Impact Sports

Laura W. Bancroft, MD[a,b,*]

KEYWORDS

- Fracture • Scapholunate ligament tear • Lunatotriquetral ligament tear
- Triangular fibrocartilage tear • DeQuervain tenosynovitis • Intersection syndrome

KEY POINTS

- Wrist injuries can be categorized as those caused by high- or low-impact sports.
- The spectrum of high-impact injuries of the wrist ranges from displaced fractures and dislocations to ligamentous and acute tendinous tears.
- Low-impact sports typically result in nondisplaced or occult fractures, contusions, stress reaction, ligamentous sprain, tendinopathy, tenosynovitis, or tendon subluxation.

INTRODUCTION

Wrist injuries can be categorized as those caused by high- or low-impact sports. Examples of high-impact sports include auto racing, motorcross or bicycle racing, in-line skating, gymnastics, football, and soccer, and winter sports such as ice skating, snowboarding, and alpine skiing (Table 1). Low-impact sports include tennis, track and field, and golf (see Table 1). The spectrum of high-impact injuries of the wrist ranges from displaced fractures and dislocations to ligamentous and acute tendinous tears (Table 2). On the other hand, low-impact sports typically result in nondisplaced or occult fractures, contusions, stress reaction, ligamentous sprain, tendinopathy, tenosynovitis, or tendon subluxation (see Table 2). Imaging modalities for detection of injuries include radiography, computed tomography (CT) magnetic resonance imaging (MRI), magnetic resonance or CT arthrography, and occasionally skeletal scintigraphy.

OSSEOUS TRAUMA
Fractures

The spectrum of osseous trauma ranges from fractures and dislocations induced by high-impact sports to contusions and stress response caused by low-impact sports. Distal radial fractures are very common injuries among athletes, and they can be sustained in both high-impact and low-impact types of activities. High-impact wrist injuries typically are intra-articular and comminuted, and they may be accompanied by lipohemarthrosis or fat in the tendon sheaths.[1] Fractures can be sustained by soccer, equestrian sports, auto racing, motorcross or bicycle racing, football, snowboarding, in-line skating, ice skating, and certain gymnastics/acrobatics maneuvers.[2–4] Ninety-six percent of wrist injuries from snowboarding are induced by a fall, and distal radial fractures are nearly twice as likely to be secondary to a backward fall than a forward fall.[3,5] However, significant reduction in wrist injuries in snowboarders and

No disclosures.

[a] University of Central Florida College of Medicine, 6850 Lake Nona Blvd, Orlando, FL 32827, USA; [b] Florida State University College of Medicine, 1115 West Call Street, Tallahassee, FL 32306, USA
* Department of Radiology, Florida Hospital, 601 E. Rollins, Orlando, FL 32803.
E-mail address: Laura.bancroft.md@flhosp.org

Radiol Clin N Am 51 (2013) 299–311
http://dx.doi.org/10.1016/j.rcl.2012.09.017

Table 1
Examples of high-impact versus low-impact sports resulting in wrist injuries

High-Impact Sports	Low-Impact Sports
Auto racing	Tennis
In-line/ice skating	Track and field
Snow boarding	Golf
Alpine skiing	Gymnastics
Motorcross/bicycle racing	Basketball
Gymnastics	
Football	
Soccer goalie	

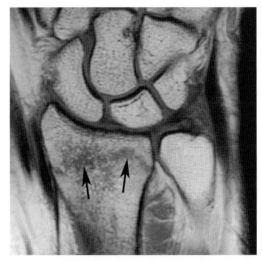

Fig. 1. Distal radial fracture. Coronal T1-weighted image through the wrist demonstrates a nondisplaced distal radial metaphyseal fracture (*arrows*) without intra-articular extension, or Frykman I fracture. This type of fracture is often seen in high-impact sports, and up to 35% of nondisplaced fractures may be overlooked on initial radiographs.

in-line skaters has been attributed to the use of wrist protectors, and experienced athletes tend to have fewer injuries.[2,6] Distal radial fractures sustained in low-impact sports are typically minimally or nondisplaced, and have been reported from falls while playing basketball or tennis or running track and field events.[7] Although radiographs are the mainstay of trauma imaging, CT may be used to further characterize the extent of fracture comminution and intra-articular extension, and MRI may help detect occult fractures (**Fig. 1**).[8,9]

Gymnast's Wrist

Gymnast's wrist is the general term used for wrist pain in gymnasts precipitated by chronic

compressive impact forces, torsional forces, and distraction.[10] These overuse injuries include distal radial physeal injury; lunate osteochondral defects; tears of the triangular fibrocartilage or scapholunate or lunatotriquetral ligaments; cartilage injury along the distal radius and carpus; and dorsal carpal ganglia.[10–12] Most commonly, however, gymnast's wrist refers to a nondisplaced, Salter-Harris type 1 physeal injury of the distal radius sustained from repetitive axial loading and hyperextension of the wrist. Floor exercise and balance beam maneuvers will direct the body's forces onto the unfused distal radial metaphyses in skeletally immature patients, resulting in widening of the physis, cystic change, and fragmentation of the adjacent metaphysic (**Fig. 2**). Pommel horse exercises in men's gymnastics can lead to distal radial stress injuries, dorsal impingement, and triangular fibrocartilage complex tears due to repetitive loading.[13] Premature closure of the distal radial physis and ulnar positive variance can be associated with gymnast's wrist.[14] Older female gymnasts are at increased risk for acute injuries of the wrist, and stress fractures are common.[15]

Scaphoid Fractures

Carpal fractures can occur with both high- and low-impact sports. The scaphoid is the most commonly fractured carpal bone, followed by the

Table 2
High-impact versus low-impact wrist injuries

High-Impact Injuries	Low-Impact Injuries
Displaced fractures (radius, scaphoid, capitate)	Fractures, nondisplaced or occult Contusions Stress reaction Complex regional pain syndrome
Dislocations (lunate, perilunate, carpometacarpal joint)	
Ligamentous tears	Ligamentous sprain
Acute tendon tear	Tendinopathy Tenosynovitis (deQuervain, extensor carpi ulnaris) Tendon subluxation (ECU)

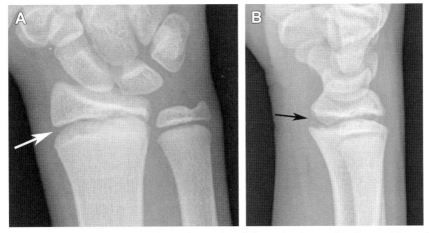

Fig. 2. Gymnast's wrist. PA (*A*) and lateral (*B*) radiographs of the wrist show widening and irregularity of the distal radial physis (*arrows*), which is more pronounced radially and volarly.

triquetrum, capitate, and lunate. Scaphoid fractures account for 60% to 70% of all carpal fractures; they occur with forced dorsiflexion and axial loading of the wrist and can be evoked by falls during a variety of sports, such as football and snowboarding. Patients clinically will present with tenderness and swelling in the anatomic snuffbox. Radiographs may be negative initially, and additional imaging is often obtained to secure a diagnosis.[16] Tomosynthesis is uncommonly used today, but it has proven to have a greater sensitivity for the detection of fracture compared with conventional radiographs.[17] Follow-up radiographs, MRI, CT, and skeletal scintigraphy are all imaging modalities that clinicians may order to detect occult fractures. Several studies have validated the benefit of MRI and the fact that it may outweigh the costs associated with lost productivity from unnecessary cast immobilization, especially in elite athletes.[16,18] Fractures in adults and most children are linear defects; however, impacted buckle fractures may occur in older children and adolescents.[19] Of note, focal carpal bony depressions are common in skeletally immature patients and should not be confused with impaction fractures.[20,21] Focused sonography, which detects cortical disruption of the scaphoid and/or effusions of the radiocarpal and scapho-trapezium-trapezoid joints may prompt further imaging with CT in patients with negative radiographs in the emergent setting.[22]

Athletes should be aware that the healing time of scaphoid fractures depends on its anatomic location, since scaphoid waist fractures can take up to 9 weeks to heal, and proximal pole injuries rarely unite before 4 months.[23] Scaphoid fractures may occur in isolation (**Fig. 3**A) or in conjunction with

other osseous or soft tissue injuries (see **Fig. 3**B). Complications of scaphoid fractures include malunion or humpback deformity caused by flexion deformity of the healing fragments (see **Fig. 3**C), nonunion in approximately 5% of fractures (see **Fig. 3**D), and avascular necrosis in a high percentage of proximal pole scaphoid fractures.[24,25] Increased radiodensity of the proximal pole fragment and absence of converging trabeculae on CT are highly suggestive of avascular necrosis and persistent nonunion.[24] Scaphoid nonunion will manifest as persistent fluid in the fracture line on MRI, with adjacent low T1- and T2-weighted marrow signal corresponding to fibrosis and sclerosis. The nonviable proximal pole fragment will fail to enhance due to its lack of vascularity.

Fracture of Hook of Hamate and Other Carpal Bones

Hook of the hamate (hamulus) fractures account for 2% of all carpal fractures, and they are endemic in sports where the hand grips the base of the club, bat or stick.[26] Golf, baseball, and hockey are common offending sports, and fractures can be caused by a check swing in baseball or grounding of a golf club. The carpal tunnel view is the best radiographic projection to detect hook of hamate fractures and delineate the size and position of the fracture fragment (**Fig. 4**A). MRI has the advantage of detecting the degree of associated soft tissue injuries and potential hematoma within the carpal tunnel (see **Fig. 4**B).[26] Other carpal bone fractures are even less common. Capitate fractures account for about 1% of all carpal fractures, occur with severe forces of a fall

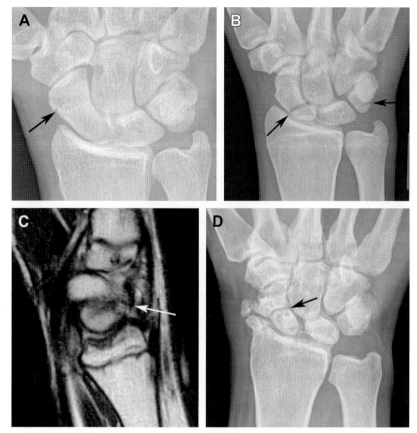

Fig. 3. Scaphoid fracture. (*A*) PA radiograph demonstrates an isolated scaphoid fracture (*arrow*) through the distal pole of the scaphoid. (*B*) Scaphoid fractures may occur in conjunction with other injuries, such as this patient with fractures through the proximal pole of the scaphoid and triquetrum (*arrows*). (*C*) Complications of scaphoid fracture include the humpback deformity (*arrow*) caused by flexion of the healing fragments, as shown on this sagittal proton density MRI. (*D*) Scaphoid nonunion (*arrow*) is another complication of scaphoid fracture, which may or may not be accompanied by avascular necrosis of the proximal pole fragment.

on an outstretched hand or direct strike against the dorsum of a flexed hand, and are often occult on radiographs. MRI has proven to be very sensitive for the detection of occult carpal bone fracture (**Fig. 5**).

Contusions

Low-impact trauma that is not forceful enough to induce a fracture can result in osseous contusions or stress reaction. Radiographs will be unrevealing, but MRI will show marrow edema-like signal

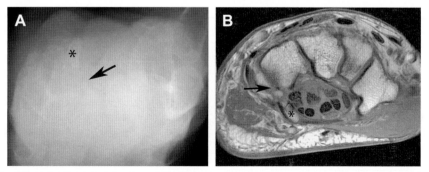

Fig. 4. Hook of hamate (hamulus) fracture. (*A*) Carpal tunnel view is the best radiographic projection to detect hook of hamate fractures (*arrow*) and delineate the size and position of the fracture fragment (*asterisk*). (*B*) MRI has the advantage of detecting the degree of associated soft tissue injuries and any hematoma within the carpal tunnel in cases of hook of hamate fracture (*arrow*).

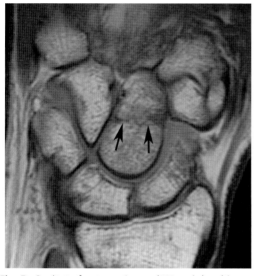

Fig. 5. Capitate fracture. Coronal T1-weighted image demonstrates a nondisplaced capitate fracture (*arrows*). Capitate fractures account for about 1% of all carpal fractures, and occur with severe forces of a fall on an outstretched hand or direct strike against the dorsum of a flexed hand.

changes without a discrete fracture line (**Fig. 6**). A clear history of trauma should be elicited from the patient, as studies have shown that asymptomatic children may also demonstrate high T2-weighted and low T1-weighted signal in at least 1 carpal bone on MRI, simulating the appearance of contusion.[21]

Dislocations

Carpal and metacarpal dislocations may occur in conjunction with fractures (**Fig. 7**) or in isolation (**Fig. 8**). Metacarpal base dislocations are almost always posterior and most commonly involve the fifth metacarpal base. Fractures of the metacarpal base and/or hamate often accompany these injuries (see **Fig. 7**). Lunate and perilunate dislocations or fracture-dislocations (see **Fig. 8**) can result from high-impact athletics such as expert snowboarding and require open reduction, ligamentous and osseous repair, and protection of the repair with supplemental fixation.[3,27] Lateral radiographs will show the volar dislocation of the lunate, called the spilled teacup sign, due to proximal rotation of the lunate about its intact palmar ligaments (see **Fig. 8**). Posteroanterior (PA) radiographs will show a widened scapholunate interval or scaphoid ring sign generated by rotation of the scaphoid with perilunate dislocation, and lateral radiographs will show loss of the colinearity of the radius, lunate, and capitate.[27,28] CT may be helpful in assessing the position and degree of comminution of the fracture, and MRI excels at detecting occult fractures, contusions, and ligamentous injuries.

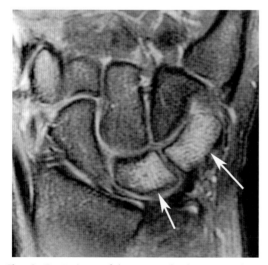

Fig. 6. Contusions of lunate and triquetrum. Low-impact trauma may result in contusions, as shown on this coronal FSE T2-weighted fat-suppressed image of lunate and triquetral contusions (*arrows*).

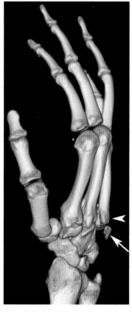

Fig. 7. Metacarpal base fracture with dorsal dislocation. 3-dimensional surface-rendered CT image of the hand demonstrates posteriorly displaced hamate fracture (*arrow*) and dorsal dislocation of the fourth and fifth metacarpal bases.

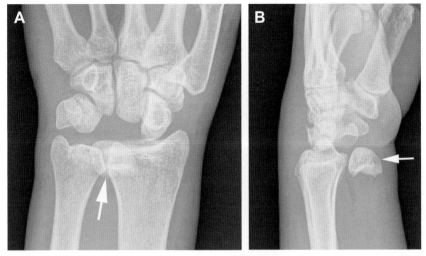

Fig. 8. Lunate dislocation. PA (A) and lateral (B) views of the wrist show volar dislocation and inversion of the lunate (arrows) due to complete disruption of the dorsal and distal ligamentous attachments. This extreme positioning of the lunate is an upside down teacup, as opposed to the more commonly tilted spilled teacup sign.

Distal Radioulnar Joint Instability

Patients with distal radioulnar joint (DRUJ) instability present with ulnar-sided wrist pain, swelling, and difficulty with gripping and forearm rotation. Subluxation or dislocation of the DRUJ is caused by failure of the triangular fibrocartilage complex (TFCC), especially the foveal insertion of the TFCC and the dorsal and volar radiolunar ligaments.[29,30] Radiographs may demonstrate concomitant ulnar styloid base fractures, widening of the DRUJ on PA radiographs, dislocation on lateral radiographs, and more than 5 mm negative ulnar variance.[31] Axial imaging with either CT or MRI (Fig. 9) can demonstrate excessive (15%–20%) dorsal translation of the ulnar head relative to the anterior-to-posterior width of the sigmoid notch of the radius when the wrist is pronated.[30] Locked dislocation of the ulnar head may be detected at the time of imaging, similar to an engaged Hill-Sachs lesion in the shoulder.[29] MRI will commonly have an associated tear of the foveal attachment of the TFC, and complex DRUJ dislocations may also show disruption of the DRUJ ligaments, portions of the interosseous membrane, extensor carpi ulnaris (ECU) tendon sheath, and ulnar styloid fracture.[20,29,32]

Complex Regional Pain Syndrome

Although it is not an intrinsic lesion of bone, complex regional pain syndrome manifests osseous changes due to trauma. Lack of autonomic regulation after relatively low-impact trauma can result in severe pain that is out of proportion to the degree of trauma. Radiographs may display osteopenia of the involved region (Fig. 10A) due to

hyperemia and washout of osseous minerals. Patients will have markedly increased radiotracer uptake (see Fig. 10B) on skeletal scintigraphy due to the regional hyperemia.

SOFT TISSUE TRAUMA
Intrinsic Ligament Tears

Ligamentous injuries of the wrist are categorized into those of the intrinsic ligaments and extrinsic ligaments. The 2 most important stabilizing intrinsic ligaments are the scapholunate (SL) and lunatotriquetral (or lunotriquetral) ligaments.[33] The SL ligament is the key stabilizer of the wrist, and tears

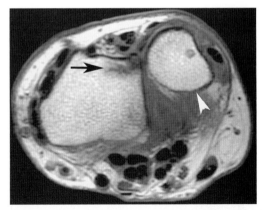

Fig. 9. Dorsal radioulnar joint instability with dorsal subluxation of the ulnar head and distal radial impaction fracture. Axial T1-weighted image of the wrist shows dorsal subluxation of the ulnar head (arrowhead) due to disruption of the volar distal radioulnar ligament (not seen) and impaction fracture (arrow) of the dorsal radius. Injuries are commonly associated with ulnar-sided triangular fibrocartilage tears.

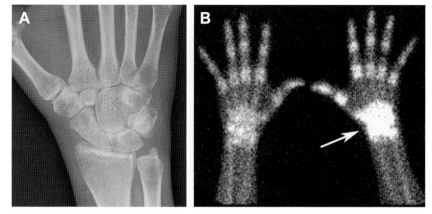

Fig. 10. Complex regional pain syndrome. (A) Lack of autonomic regulation after relatively low-impact trauma can result in severe pain that is out of proportion to the degree of trauma and osteopenia due to hyperemia and washout of minerals. (B) Patients will have markedly increased radiotracer uptake (*arrow*) on skeletal scintigraphy due to hyperemia in this disorder.

result in the most common form of carpal instability. The SL ligament is comprised of bandlike dorsal and volar components, and a triangular-shaped proximal (membranous) component; the dorsal component is twice as thick as the volar component.[34] Tears result from falls on a pronated, outstretched hand (commonly with football) or excessive force applied to a hyperextended wrist during a fall. Noncontact sports (ie, baseball, basketball, and soccer) may result in SL tears.[23] Patients will complain of dorsal wrist pain, swelling, popping sounds with wrist motion, and weakness; symptoms are aggravated by provocative wrist motion and resistance (Rosner).[23] MRI yields 89% sensitivity for the detection of SL ligament tears, whereas magnetic resonance arthrography

raises the sensitivity to 100% (**Fig. 11A**).[35,36] SL ligament tears may result in widening of the SL interval more than 3 mm (see **Fig. 11B**) and loss of the normal carpal alignment. Dorsal intercalated segmental instability (DISI) caused by SL ligament disruption causes dorsal tilt of the lunate and increased capitate-lunate angle greater than 30° (see **Fig. 11C**).[37,38] Caution should be exercised when diagnosing DISI deformity on MRI, since false-positive results may occur due to non-neutral wrist positioning.[39] CT arthrography is an excellent alternative to MRI, when MRI is contraindicated or not available.[40,41]

The lunatotriquetral (LT) ligament, similar to the SL ligament, also has bandlike volar and dorsal components and a triangular-shaped membranous

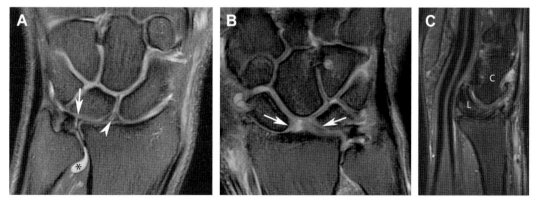

Fig. 11. Scapholunate ligament tear. (A) Coronal FSE T2-weighted fat-suppressed image shows a linear tear of the scapholunate ligament (*arrowhead*) as well as a tear through the radial aspect of the TFC (*arrow*). Fluid extends through the full-thickness TFC tear into the distal radioulnar joint (*asterisk*). (B) Scapholunate ligament tear is associated with widening of the SL interval (*arrows*). (C) Although lateral radiographs are more accurate for assessing the degree of DISI deformity, sagittal MR imaging can show the dorsal tilt of the lunate (L) relative to the radius and capitate (C).

component. The volar portion of the LT ligament is the strongest and thickest, and has contributions from the ulnocapitate ligament.[34] LT ligament tears are 6 times less common than SL ligament tears, and they are caused by loading forces while the wrist is in maximal extension, or radial deviation of the wrist with or without pronation.[34] However, unlike SL ligament tears, tearing of the LT ligament usually does not result in joint space widening between the 2 bones. MRI is less accurate for detecting LT ligament tears compared with SL tears, with 82% sensitivity and 100% specificity (**Fig. 12**); however, magnetic resonance arthrography raises the sensitivity to 100%.[35] LT ligament tearing may be the result of end-stage perilunate instability or associated with ulnocarpal abutment syndrome.[39]

Extrinsic Ligament Tears

There are multiple volar and dorsal extrinsic ligaments of the wrist, and they are named after their osseous attachments. The radioscaphocapitate ligament is the most important of the volar ligaments, and the volar radiolunotriquetral ligament (or long radiolunate ligament) is the largest and an important stabilizer. The ulnolunate and ulnotriquetral ligaments comprise a portion of the triangular fibrocartilage complex, and the primary dorsal stabilizer is the dorsal radiocarpal ligament.[42] Midcarpal instability is a nondissociative carpal instability caused by a variety of extrinsic ligament injuries.[43] Extrinsic ligament injuries are

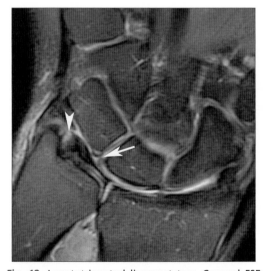

Fig. 12. Lunatotriquetral ligament tear. Coronal FSE T2-weighted fat-suppressed image shows tearing of the LT ligament (*arrow*) as well as the ulnar aspect of the TFC (*arrowhead*).

best detected with magnetic resonance arthrography (and to a lesser extent conventional MRI), but sensitivities are less than those of intrinsic ligaments.[44] In 1 study of arthroscopically proven cases of radioscaphocapitate and long radiolunate tears, 63% and 25% sensitivities and 56% and 67% specificities were reported, respectively.[45] Longitudinal split tears of the ulnotriquetral ligament have been reported, in which patients present with pain, but no instability of the DRUJ or ulnocarpal joint.[46] Three-dimensional fast-spin echo (FSE) cube imaging of the wrist obtained in the coronal plane has shown improved signal-to-noise ratio and less blurring artifact compared with conventional 2-dimensional FSE imaging, and it is becoming more widely used.[47]

Triangular Fibrocartilage Tears

The triangular fibrocartilage complex (TFCC) is comprised of the triangular fibrocartilage (TFC) disc, the meniscal homolog, ulnar collateral ligament, dorsal and volar radioulnar ligaments, subsheath of the ECU tendon, and ulnocarpal and triangular ligaments.[34,41] The disc is composed of 2 laminae that both attach laterally to the distal radius (the proximal one is attached to the fovea by the upper lamina of the triangular ligament; the distal one attaches to the tip of the ulnar styloid by the lower lamina of the triangular ligament), and there is a hyperintense space between the 2 bands, called the ligamentum subcruentum.[34,48] Patients with TFC tears complain of pain with pronation/supination and loading of the extended wrist, catching, and snapping. The Palmer classification categorizes TFCC tears into traumatic (type 1) and degenerative (type 2) subtypes.[49] Type 1A lesions are isolated central disc perforations; type 1B lesions are peripheral ulnar-sided tears (which may be associated with ulnar styloid fractures). Type 1C lesions are distal TFCC disruptions (from ulnocarpal ligaments), and type 1D lesions are radial-sided disruptions (often associated with sigmoid notch fracture).[49]

MRI is an accurate imaging modality for the detection TFCC tears, with 91% accuracy reported in 1 series using 3 T strength magnets and 83% accuracy with 1.5 T magnets (**Fig. 13**A).[50] MRI can detect partial-thickness tearing of the radial, central, or ulnar attachments and complex tearing and bucket-handle tears.[51] Magnetic resonance arthrography with radiocarpal joint injection allows for superior contrast resolution and joint distention and has sensitivities up to 100% for the detection of TFCC tears.[35] A meta-analysis of 21 studies spanning the past

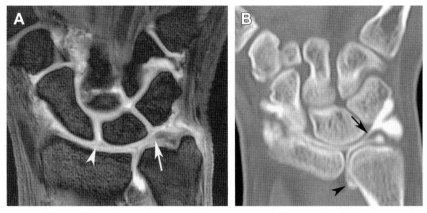

Fig. 13. Triangular fibrocartilage tear. (*A*) magnetic resonance arthrography delineates contrast extension through the TFC (*arrow*) and SL ligament (*arrowhead*) tears, with communication of injected contrast into the DRUJ and midcarpal joints. (*B*) CT arthrography shows the retracted full-thickness tear of the radial attachment of the TFC (*arrow*), with communication of contrast into the distal radioulnar joint (*arrowhead*).

2 decades revealed an overall 84% sensitivity and 95% specificity for TFC tears using magnetic resonance arthrography, although accuracy rates have increased with newer equipment and 3 T magnets.[52,53] Ulnar-sided tears are more difficult to appreciate on conventional MRI due to the increased signal and striated appearance of the triangular ligament; however, magnetic resonance arthrography has been shown to increase accuracy.[48,54] Of note, abnormalities of the TFCC in asymptomatic patients is common (39 of 103 patients in 1 study), and lesions increase in patients older than 50 years of age.[55] CT arthrography after radiocarpal injection of contrast is nearly as sensitive in detecting full-thickness or distal partial-thickness tears of the TFC (see Fig. 13B); partial thickness proximal TFC tears will not be detected with CT arthrography unless distal radioulnar injection is performed. CT arthrography excels in detecting small flake fractures from the fovea that might be overlooked with MRI.[41] Sonography also has received more attention in the literature for the evaluating injuries of the triangular fibrocartilage and intrinsic and extrinsic ligaments of the wrist.[56]

TENDON INJURIES

Tendon failure is caused by tendon overload in the athlete, and it can be the result of faulty training techniques, incorrect training program/equipment, and/or an abrupt increase in training intensity. High-impact trauma can result in acute tendon tears (Figs. 14 and 15), whereas low-impact, repetitive trauma renders shear stresses across the tendons as they move across static structures in confined spaces. These stresses can lead to

a cascade of tenosynovitis, tendinopathy, and eventually tendon tear.

ECU Tendon Injuries

ECU tendinopathy and tendon tears occur with repetitive wrist motion, usually in racquet sports. With 2-handed backhand, the nondominant wrist will undergo exaggerated ulnar deviation, and the patient may complain of tenderness over the sixth extensor compartment adjacent to the ulnar styloid (see Fig. 14). The golf casting maneuver is the incorrect, premature wrist release on the downswing that can lead to ECU pathology. The ECU tendon can also sublux if there is traumatic rupture of the ECU subsheath caused by forceful supination of the forearm, flexion, and ulnar deviation of the wrist during tennis, baseball or other racquet sports. The ECU will become perched on

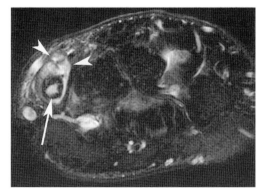

Fig. 14. ECU tendon tear. Axial FSE T2-weighted fat-suppressed image shows high-grade partial-thickness tearing of the ECU (*arrow*) with hemorrhage in the surrounding tendon sheath (*arrowheads*).

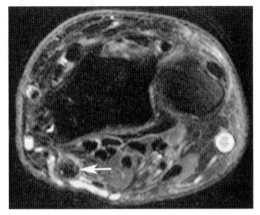

Fig. 15. Flexor carpi radialis tendon tear. Axial FSE T2-weighted fat-suppressed image shows high-grade partial-thickness tearing of the flexor carpi radialis (*arrow*) with hemorrhage in the surrounding tendon sheath.

the intertubercular groove, cause painful snapping and clicking, and may mimic DRUJ instability.[57] Injuries are best detected with sonography or MRI while eliciting the provocative maneuver.[39,58]

Flexor Carpi Radialis Tendon Injuries

Flexor tendon injuries are common in racquet sports and golf. With golf, the trailing hand normally undergoes a wider range or flexion and extension during the swing. In addition, unwanted fat shots and divots impart large forces onto the wrist. The spectrum of flexor carpi radialis tendon injuries ranges from tendinopathy (with tenderness over the insertion onto the second metacarpal base and pain with resisted wrist flexion), to rupture with inability of the patient to flex the wrist (see **Fig. 15**).

DeQuervain Tenosynovitis

DeQuervain tenosynovitis is the most common tendinopathy of the wrist in athletes, and it is caused by shear stress injury of the first extensor compartment tendons along the radial styloid. Acute sprains and chronic overuse in golf and racquet sports occur from forceful grasping of the club in ulnar deviation. Repetitive wrist motion with radial/ulnar deviation and flexion/extension can cause tenosynovitis or tendon tearing of the extensor pollicis brevis and abductor pollicis longus tendons, and this is easily detected with MRI (**Fig. 16**).

Intersection Syndrome

There are 2 types of intersection syndrome described in the literature. The classic intersection syndrome is an overuse disorder caused by

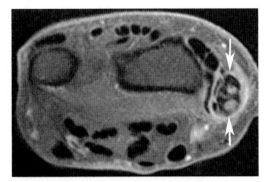

Fig. 16. DeQuervain tenosynovitis. Axial proton density image shows split tears of the enlarged extensor pollicis brevis and abductor pollicis longus tendons (*arrows*) along the distal radius.

low-impact trauma, also known as oarsmen's wrist, squeaker's wrist, or crossover syndrome.[59] Rowing, canoeing, racquet sports, horseback riding, and skiing have all been reported as causes of intersection syndrome.[59] MRI is useful in detecting peritendinous edema around the first and second extensor compartment tendons in the distal forearm as they cross over each other (**Fig. 17**). In contradistinction, distal intersection syndrome results in dorsal hand edema-like signal changes of the second and third extensor compartment tendons as they cross over each other. This specific form of tenosynovitis occurs because of the confined tendons, biomechanical pulley effect exerted by Lister tubercle, and constraining effect of the extensor retinaculum (**Fig. 18**).[60]

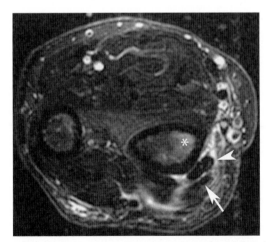

Fig. 17. Intersection syndrome. Axial FSE T2-weighted fat-suppressed image shows peritendinous edema around the first (*arrowhead*) and second (*arrow*) extensor compartment tendons in the distal forearm as they cross over each other. Notice the reactive marrow edema-like signal changes in the subjacent distal radius (*asterisk*).

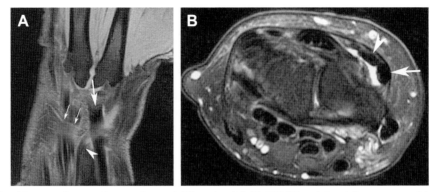

Fig. 18. Distal intersection syndrome. Coronal (*A*) and axial (*B*) FSE T2-weighted fat-suppressed images show edema-like signal changes of the second and third extensor compartment tendons as they cross over each other in the dorsum of the hand and are confined by the biomechanical pulley effect exerted by Lister tubercle and the constraining effect of the extensor retinaculum. (extensor carpi radialis tendon = large arrows, extensor pollicis longus = arrowheads, extensor retinaculum = small arrows).

SUMMARY

In conclusion, sports-related wrist injuries may be sustained during a variety of high- or low-impact activities, and the severity of osseous and/or soft tissue injury will reflect the severity of transmitted force. Displaced fractures and carpal dislocations are more common in motorized or high-velocity sports, detected with radiography, and most commonly involve the radius and scaphoid. Sports that transmit less energy to the wrist will cause less severe injuries (such as contusions or stress reactions), and additional higher-level imaging may be required to make the diagnosis. Ligamentous and tendinous injuries of the wrist range from tendinopathy and tenosynovitis with repetitive, low-impact sports all the way to acute rupture with high-impact energy. These soft tissue injuries are best delineated with MRI or magnetic resonance arthrography, but they may also be detected with other modalities such as CT arthrography, sonography, or skeletal scintigraphy.

REFERENCES

1. Le Corroller T, Parratte S, Zink JV, et al. Floating fat in the wrist joint and in the tendon sheaths. Skeletal Radiol 2010;39(9):931–3.
2. Barr LV, Imam S, Crawford JR, et al. Skating on thin ice: a study of the injuries sustained at a temporary ice skating rink. Int Orthop 2010;34(5):743–6.
3. Idzikowski JR, Janes PC, Abbott PJ. Upper extremity snowboarding injuries: ten-year results from the Colorado Snowboard Injury Survey. Am J Sports Med 2000;28(6):825–31.
4. Carmont MR, Daynes R, Sedgwick DM. The impact of an extreme sports event on a district general hospital. Scott Med J 2005;50(3):106–8.
5. Schmitt KU, Wider D, Michel FI, et al. Characterizing the mechanical parameters of forward and backward falls as experienced in snowboarding. Sports Biomech 2012;11(1):57–72.
6. Burkhart TA, Andrews DM. The effectiveness of wrist guards for reducing wrist and elbow accelerations resulting from simulated forward falls. J Appl Biomech 2010;26(3):281–9.
7. Flood L, Harrison JE. Epidemiology of basketball and netball injuries that resulted in hospital admission in Australia, 2000-2004. Med J Aust 2009;190(2):87–90.
8. Goldfarb CA, Yin Y, Gilula LA, et al. Wrist fractures: what the clinician wants to know. Radiology 2001; 219(1):11–28.
9. Geijer M, El-Khoury GY. MDCT in the evaluation of skeletal trauma: principles, protocols, and clinical applications. Emerg Radiol 2006;13(1):7–18.
10. Webb BG, Rettig LA. Gymnastic wrist injuries. Curr Sports Med Rep 2008;7(5):289–95.
11. Davis KW. Imaging pediatric sports injuries: upper extremity. Radiol Clin North Am 2010;48(6):1199–211.
12. Dwek JR, Cardoso F, Chung CB. MR imaging of overuse injuries in the skeletally immature gymnast: spectrum of soft-tissue and osseous lesions in the hand and wrist. Pediatr Radiol 2009;39(12):1310–6.
13. Fujihara T, Gervais P. Circles with a suspended aid: reducing pommel reaction forces. Sports Biomech 2012;11(1):34–47.
14. Hogan KA, Gross RH. Overuse injuries in pediatric athletes. Orthop Clin North Am 2003;34(3):405–15.
15. O'Kane JW, Levy MR, Pietila KE, et al. Survey of injuries in Seattle area levels 4 to 10 female club gymnasts. Clin J Sport Med 2011;21(6):486–92.
16. Mallee W, Doornberg JN, Ring D, et al. Comparison of CT and MRI for diagnosis of suspected scaphoid fractures. J Bone Joint Surg Am 2011;93(1):20–8.
17. Ottenin MA, Jacquot A, Grospretre O, et al. Evaluation of the diagnostic performance of tomosynthesis

in fractures of the wrist. AJR Am J Roentgenol 2012; 198(1):180–6.

18. Khalid M, Jummani ZR, Kanagaraj K, et al. Role of MRI in the diagnosis of clinically suspected scaphoid fracture: analysis of 611 consecutive cases and literature review. Emerg Med J 2010; 27(4):266–9.

19. Swischuk LE. Skeletal trauma in children: what is different? Injury to wrist in a ten-year-old boy. Emerg Radiol 2008;15(5):343–4.

20. Avenarius DM, Ording Müller LS, Eldevik P, et al. The paediatric wrist revisited-findings of bony depressions in healthy children on radiographs compared to MRI. Pediatr Radiol 2012;42(7):791–8.

21. Ording Müller LS, Avenarius D, Damasio B, et al. The paediatric wrist revisited: redefining MR findings in healthy children. Ann Rheum Dis 2011; 70(4):605–10.

22. Platon A, Poletti PA, Van Aaken J, et al. Occult fractures of the scaphoid: the role of ultrasonography in the emergency department. Skeletal Radiol 2011; 40(7):869–75.

23. Rosner JL, Zlatkin MB, Clifford P, et al. Imaging of athletic wrist and hand injuries. Semin Musculoskelet Radiol 2004;8(1):57–79.

24. Smith ML, Bain GI, Chabrel N, et al. Using computed tomography to assist with diagnosis of avascular necrosis complicating chronic scaphoid nonunion. J Hand Surg Am 2009;34(6):1037–43.

25. Deady LH, Salonen D. Skiing and snowboarding injuries: a review with a focus on mechanism of injury. Radiol Clin North Am 2010;48(6):1113–24.

26. Pierre-Jerome C, Moncayo V, Terk MR. The Guyon's canal in perspective: 3-T MRI assessment of the normal anatomy, the anatomical variations and the Guyon's canal syndrome. Surg Radiol Anat 2011; 33(10):897–903.

27. Stanbury SJ, Elfar JC. Perilunate dislocation and perilunate fracture-dislocation. J Am Acad Orthop Surg 2011;19(9):554–62.

28. Kannikeswaran N, Sethuraman U. Lunate and perilunate dislocations. Pediatr Emerg Care 2010;26(12): 921–4.

29. Mulford JS, Axelrod TS. Traumatic injuries of the distal radioulnar joint. Hand Clin 2010;26(1):155–63.

30. Ehman EC, Hayes ML, Berger RA, et al. Subluxation of the distal radioulnar joint as a predictor of foveal triangular fibrocartilage complex tears. J Hand Surg Am 2011;36(11):1780–4.

31. Garrigues GE, Sabesan V, Aldridge JM 3rd. Acute distal radioulnar joint instability. J Surg Orthop Adv 2008;17(4):262–6.

32. Amrami KK, Moran SL, Berger RA, et al. Imaging the distal radioulnar joint. Hand Clin 2010;26(4): 467–75.

33. Stein JM, Cook TS, Simonson S, et al. Normal and variant anatomy of the wrist and hand on MR imaging. Magn Reson Imaging Clin N Am 2011; 19(3):595–608.

34. Burns JE, Tanaka T, Ueno T, et al. Pitfalls that may mimic injuries of the triangular fibrocartilage and proximal intrinsic wrist ligaments at MR imaging. Radiographics 2011;31(1):63–78.

35. Magee T. Comparison of 3-T MRI and arthroscopy of intrinsic wrist ligament and TFCC tears. AJR Am J Roentgenol 2009;192:8–85.

36. van Dijke CF, Wiarda BM. High resolution wrist MR arthrography at 1.5T. JBR-BTR 2009;92(1):53–9.

37. Pliefke J, Stengel D, Rademacher G, et al. Diagnostic accuracy of plain radiographs and cineradiography in diagnosing traumatic scapholunate dissociation. Skeletal Radiol 2008;37(2):139–45.

38. Picha BM, Konstantakos EK, Gordon DA. Incidence of bilateral scapholunate dissociation in symptomatic and asymptomatic wrists. J Hand Surg Am 2012;37(6):1130–5.

39. Malone WJ, Snowden R, Alvi F, et al. Pitfalls of wrist MR imaging. Magn Reson Imaging Clin N Am 2010; 18(4):643–62.

40. Ramdhian-Wihlm R, Le Minor JM, Schmittbuhl M, et al. Cone-beam computed tomography arthrography: an innovative modality for the evaluation of wrist ligament and cartilage injuries. Skeletal Radiol 2012; 41(8):963–9.

41. Cerezal L, de Dios Berná-Mestre J, Canga A, et al. MR and CT arthrography of the wrist. Semin Musculoskelet Radiol 2012;16(1):27–41.

42. Davis KW, Blankenbaker DG. Imaging the ligaments and tendons of the wrist. Semin Roentgenol 2010; 45(3):194–217.

43. Toms AP, Chojnowski A, Cahir JG. Midcarpal instability: a radiological perspective. Skeletal Radiol 2011;40(5):533–41.

44. Shahabpour M, De Maeseneer M, Pouders C, et al. MR imaging of normal extrinsic wrist ligaments using thin slices with clinical and surgical correlation. Eur J Radiol 2011;77(2):196–201.

45. Mak WH, Szabo RM, Myo GK. Assessment of volar radiocarpal ligaments: MR arthrographic and arthroscopic correlation. AJR Am J Roentgenol 2012; 198(2):423–7.

46. Tay SC, Berger RA, Parker WL. Longitudinal split tears of the ulnotriquetral ligament. Hand Clin 2010;26(4):495–501.

47. Stevens KJ, Wallace CG, Chen W, et al. Imaging of the wrist at 1.5 Tesla using isotropic three-dimensional fast spin echo cube. J Magn Reson Imaging 2011;33(4):908–15.

48. Yoshioka H, Burns JE. Magnetic resonance imaging of triangular fibrocartilage. J Magn Reson Imaging 2012;35(4):764–78.

49. Palmer AK. Triangular fibrocartilage complex lesions: a classification. J Hand Surg Am 1989; 14(4):594–606.

50. Anderson ML, Skinner JA, Felmlee JP, et al. Diagnostic comparison of 1.5 Tesla and 3.0 Tesla preoperative MRI of the wrist in patients with ulnar-sided wrist pain. J Hand Surg Am 2008; 33(7):1153–9.

51. Theumann N, Kamel EM, Bollmann C, et al. Bucket-handle tear of the triangular fibrocartilage complex: case report of a complex peripheral injury with separation of the distal radioulnar ligaments from the articular disc. Skeletal Radiol 2011;40(12):1617–21.

52. Smith TO, Drew B, Toms AP, et al. Diagnostic accuracy of magnetic resonance imaging and magnetic resonance arthrography for triangular fibrocartilaginous complex injury: a systematic review and meta-analysis. J Bone Joint Surg Am 2012;94(9):824–32.

53. Chhabra A, Soldatos T, Thawait GK, et al. Current perspectives on the advantages of 3-T MR imaging of the wrist. Radiographics 2012;32(3):879–96.

54. Rüegger C, Schmid MR, Pfirrmann CW, et al. Peripheral tear of the triangular fibrocartilage: depiction with MR arthrography of the distal radioulnar joint. AJR Am J Roentgenol 2007;188(1):187–92.

55. Iordache SD, Rowan R, Garvin GJ, et al. Prevalence of triangular fibrocartilage complex abnormalities on MRI scans of asymptomatic wrists. J Hand Surg Am 2012;37(1):98–103.

56. Taljanovic MS, Goldberg MR, Sheppard JE, et al. US of the intrinsic and extrinsic wrist ligaments and triangular fibrocartilage complex–normal anatomy and imaging technique. Radiographics 2011;31(1): e44.

57. Jeantroux J, Becce F, Guerini H, et al. Athletic injuries of the extensor carpi ulnaris subsheath: MRI findings and utility of gadolinium-enhanced fat-saturated T1-weighted sequences with wrist pronation and supination. Eur Radiol 2011;21(1): 160–6.

58. Jamadar DA, Jacobson JA, Caoili EM, et al. Musculoskeletal sonography technique: focused versus comprehensive evaluation. AJR Am J Roentgenol 2008;190(1):5–9.

59. Lee RP, Hatem SF, Recht MP. Extended MRI findings of intersection syndrome. Skeletal Radiol 2009; 38(2):157–63.

60. Parellada AJ, Gopez AG, Morrison WB, et al. Distal intersection tenosynovitis of the wrist: a lesser-known extensor tendinopathy with characteristic MR imaging features. Skeletal Radiol 2007;36(3): 203–8.

Imaging of Football Injuries to the Upper Extremity

Martin L. Lazarus, MD[a,b],*

KEYWORDS

- Football injury • Upper extremity • Imaging

KEY POINTS

- Familiarity with mechanisms of injury, position of the player, and the need for rapid diagnosis and reporting will help radiologists with imaging of football players.
- Although plain radiographs are typically the first imaging modality used, magnetic resonance imaging has become the cornerstone on which diagnoses and treatment decisions are based.
- As football athletes become stronger, faster, and more skilled, the ability to accurately assess their injuries becomes even more important, and understanding the challenges that these patients present becomes critical.

INTRODUCTION

American football is a contact sport that involves cutting and pivoting and high-speed collisions on virtually every play; this holds true for training and practice, in addition to games. Over the years, and particularly within the past 5 years, many rules and equipment changes have decreased the frequency and extent of the injuries incurred by athletes at all levels of play.

More than 1.5 million athletes play competitive football annually in the United States, at all levels of competition.[1,2] These athletes sustain 0.6 to 1.2 million injuries annually,[3,4] with any player having a 50% chance of incurring an injury during the year.[1,3–5] Patterns and frequency of injury have changed over time as the rules, equipment, and strategies have evolved. The size, speed, and fitness of the athletes has also had an effect on the patterns and frequency of injuries, particularly at the collegiate and professional levels, because players have become larger, faster, and better conditioned.

Different factors have been correlated with an increased risk of injury, including player position, with the positions handling the ball most often (quarterbacks and running backs) and, on the defensive side, those creating the greatest energy before contact (linebackers and defensive backs) having the highest risk.[1,6,7] Most injuries occur in the third quarter of a game, in the first half of the season, especially muscle strains, in which large muscle groups, such as the quadriceps and hamstrings, experience fatigue and tend to wear down early in the season.

Medical imaging has attained a preeminent role in the treatment of these athletes. Although history and physical examinations remain the primary means of diagnosis, and plain radiographs are often the first line of imaging for these players, magnetic resonance (MR) imaging has become the definitive imaging examination, particularly as the level of player becomes more elite. MR imaging is relied on by players, coaches, and team physicians because of its ability to confirm suspected diagnoses, add additional unknown information, and provide a roadmap for surgical or conservative treatment planning.

When dealing with professional football players, rapid diagnosis of an injury can be critical. The

a Department of Radiology, Evanston Hospital, Northshore University Healthsystem, 2650 Ridge Avenue, Evanston, IL 60201, USA; b The University of Chicago, Pritzker School of Medicine, 924 East 57th Street, Suite 104, Chicago, IL 60637-5415, USA
* Department of Radiology, Evanston Hospital, Northshore University Healthsystem, 2650 Ridge Avenue, Evanston, IL 60201.
E-mail address: MLazarus@northshore.org

Radiol Clin N Am 51 (2013) 313–330
http://dx.doi.org/10.1016/j.rcl.2012.11.002
0033-8389/13/$ – see front matter © 2013 Elsevier Inc. All rights reserved.

athletes' ability to compete, and compete safely at a high level, is of paramount importance. The athletes' livelihood depends on accurate results, as does the team's success. Finally, the added pressure of media and public interest in these athletes necessitates timely, accurate diagnosis. For all of these reasons, MR imaging has surpassed all other modalities when treating professional football players.

This article focuses on many of the most frequent injuries involving the upper extremity, and some less commonly described entities. Mechanisms of injury are discussed whenever possible to help in understanding the imaging findings. MR imaging is the focus for the reasons described earlier.

MR imaging protocols and sequences are only directly addressed when they do not overlap with other articles in this issue or when a sport-specific protocol must be used.

SHOULDER INJURIES

Shoulder injuries are the fourth most common musculoskeletal injury encountered in American football players. Kaplan and colleagues[8] evaluated 336 elite collegiate American football players invited to the National Football League (NFL) Combine and found that 50% had a history of shoulder injuries. The most common of these were acromioclavicular separation (41%), anterior instability (20%), rotator cuff injury (12%), clavicle fracture (4%), and posterior instability (4%). Quarterbacks and defensive backs more commonly sustained shoulder injuries. Linebackers and linemen underwent more surgical procedures, whereas anterior instability was more common in defensive players. Linemen experienced more rotator cuff injuries and posterior instability.

Rule changes prohibiting the use of the head as an initial contact point for tackling and blocking were instituted in the NFL in 1976. Since then, the shoulder has become the initial contact point used by the defensive players. Although shoulder pads may dissipate some of the forces, they do not protect against all of the compressive forces. This fact is borne out in the high number of acromioclavicular injuries.[3] A component of superimposed traumatic cuff impingement often occurs with the injuries, because the force typically drives the humerus into the acromion and coracoacromial arch, causing compression of the cuff.[3]

Rotator Cuff Lesions

In general, although the rotator cuff is more often problematic for athletes involved with overhead throwing and repetitive microtrauma, acute traumatic tears can occur in football players of all levels. Neer[9] originally described rotator cuff injury as a continuum. In athletes younger than 25 years who perform repetitive overhead activity, edema and hemorrhage initially accumulate within the subacromial space. As the rotator cuff injury evolves, fibrosis and tendinosis ensue, usually in athletes between ages 25 and 40 years. Finally, partial- and full-thickness tears develop in athletes older than 40 years. The initial stages described earlier are termed *stage I* and *II*, whereas rotator cuff tears are termed *stage III*, and often are the sequelae of subacromial space abnormalities.[9]

Rotator Cuff Injuries in the Quarterback

The mechanics of throwing for the quarterback are similar to those for a baseball pitcher. There are, however, several important differences because of the increased weight of a football relative to a baseball (15 vs 5 oz). Because of this weight discrepancy, maximal internal velocities are much less when throwing a football, as much as 3.0 to 4.5 times slower, than when throwing a baseball, and elbow extension velocities are between 2 and 3 times slower.[1,10–13] In addition, because of the increased weight, quarterbacks lead more prominently with their elbow. This flexed position shortens the lever arm, decreasing the load on the shoulder. The more erect position of the body when throwing the ball, and the decreased contribution from the trunk and legs also help decrease arm velocity. Lastly, to avoid an oncoming pass rush, quarterbacks finish their follow-through in a more erect position than a baseball pitcher. All of these factors diminish total forces acting on the shoulder of a quarterback, with a much lower incidence of rotator cuff injuries related to overuse compared with baseball pitchers.

Instead, quarterbacks (as do players of other positions) experience an inordinate amount of acute trauma to the rotator cuff compared with other athletes. Rotator cuff contusions, acute tendinopathy, or tears are seen, which usually occur because of direct trauma from contact with either another player or the ground, in the form of an axial force at the elbow with an adducted arm driving the humerus into the acromion.[11]

Blevins and colleagues[14] looked at a group of 10 football players with rotator cuff lesions and found that 5 had partial-thickness tears, 3 full-thickness tears, and 2 contusions. Gorse and colleagues[15] described an acute, traumatic supraspinatus tear in a collegiate football player, resulting from a single, compressive force as opposed to repetitive microtrauma. This athlete fell on the turf, with his elbow making initial contact.

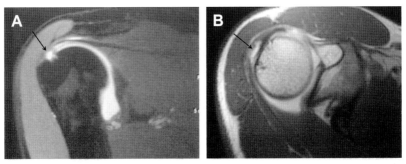

Fig. 1. Partial-thickness articular surface infraspinatus tear in a 30-year-old National Football League quarterback with increasing pain and weakness while throwing. (*A*) Oblique coronal T$_1$ MR arthrographic fat-suppressed image and (*B*) axial T$_1$-weighted non–fat-suppressed image show imbibation of contrast material within the undersurface of the anterior supraspinatus tendon (*arrow*).

The diagnostic value of MR imaging lies in its ability to differentiate cuff strain/contusion from chronic tendinosis or partial- and full-thickness tears (**Fig. 1**). MR imaging has a greater than 95% sensitivity and specificity for full-thickness tears.[16] Size of the tear has been found to be the most important prognostic factor, and the accuracy of MR imaging in assessing tear dimensions has been very good relative to surgical findings.[17] Cuff repairs are usually performed for full-thickness tears or partial-thickness tears greater than 50% of tendon thickness. Debridement is performed for tears less than 50% of tendon thickness.[1,5]

Anterior Instability

Shoulder instability is a common condition among athletes and is the most frequent sequela of traumatic dislocation. The glenohumeral joint is the most commonly dislocated major joint in the body. Although both anterior and posterior instability can occur, more than 90% of all cases of traumatic instability are anterior.

Patients with instability experience lesions to the capsulolabral mechanism. The critical lesion is detachment of the anterior labrum and capsule from the anterior glenoid, as originally described by Bankart.[18,19] Other capsular structures, including the subscapularis muscles and tendon and the anterior glenoid capsule and periosteum, may be stretched or torn (**Fig. 2**). Focal glenoid hypoplasia or aplasia may also contribute to instability.

The predominant osseous abnormality involved is the Hill-Sachs defect, which is a notch-like defect in the posterolateral humeral head resulting from encroachment of the articular surface of the humerus on the anteroinferior rim of the glenoid fossa.[18]

Treatment of shoulder instability involves either nonoperative management or surgical stabilization. Recurrence rates for nonathletes younger than 40 years with first-time dislocation is very high: between 60% and 90%.[19] In the pediatric age group, the rate may approach 95%.[20,21] If stabilization is performed in the nonathlete, recurrence rates decrease to 7% to 23%. In collision athletes, this rate increases to between 28% and 67%.[22–26]

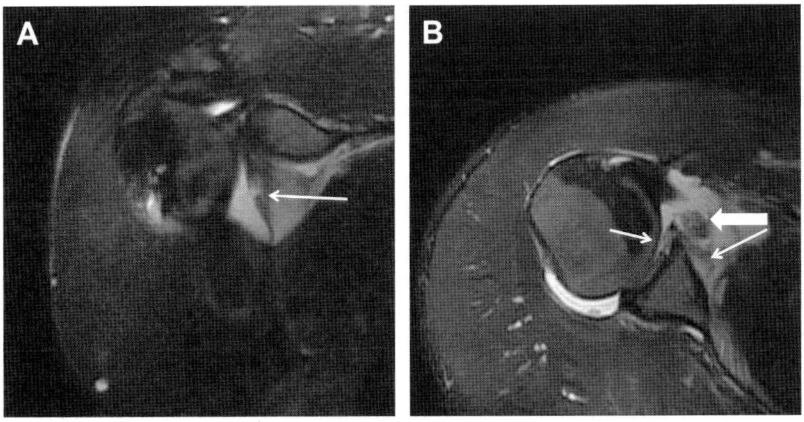

Fig. 2. Torn anterior labrum with anterior periosteal stripping and disruption of the middle glenohumeral ligament (MGHL). (*A*) Torn anterior labrum and chondral defect (*short, thin arrow*) with avulsed glenoid periosteum (*long, thin arrow*) and markedly thickened MGHL (*thick arrow*). (*B*) Tear in the anterior capsule (*arrow*).

Brophy and colleagues[27] evaluated at 42 college football players at the NFL predraft combine and found that almost 10% had a history of shoulder instability. Shoulder stabilization was the fourth most common procedure among all athletes at the combine, and this study showed that a history of shoulder stabilization shortens the expected career of a professional football player. This finding is particularly true for linemen and linebackers, who played more than 30% fewer games and years than controls did. No statistical difference was seen in career length in other position players with a history of stabilization. This discrepancy may be related to linemen and linebackers frequently placing their shoulders in extreme abduction and external rotation when pass rushing. Offensive lineman may be at risk while run and pass blocking, or during collisions with the defensive linemen.[28]

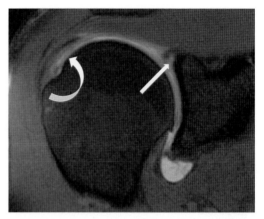

Fig. 3. Posterior superior labral tear with partial-thickness posterior supraspinatus tear in this NFL lineman with clinical instability. Coronal oblique T_1-weighted fat-saturated MR arthrographic image shows contrast material within the base of the posterior-superior labrum (*arrow*) and articular surface of the distal posterior supraspinatus tendon (*curved arrow*).

Posterior Labral Lesions and Instability

Football players are 15 times more likely to have a posterior labral lesion on MR arthrography than nonfootball players.[29,30] The difficulty in diagnosing these athletes arises from the low frequency of actual posterior instability at clinical examination. Often these athletes present with posterior pain only, creating a diagnostic dilemma.[13] High-quality MR arthrography examinations are critical in these patients. At the authors' institution, MR arthrography is the standard for elite athletes when a posterior labral abnormality is suspected.

Significant structural differences are seen between the anterior and posterior glenohumeral joint, with resultant differences in instability patterns. The posterior labrum is loosely attached to the capsule without the same ligamentous support that the anterior labrum receives.[31] Therefore, posterior labral detachment is thought to not necessarily be associated with posterior instability unless a posterior capsular lesion has occurred (**Fig. 3**).[32] This posterior capsular lesion may involve capsulolabral detachment, capsular laxity, or rotator interval lesions.[33,34]

In 1981, the National Collegiate Athletic Association implemented a rules change allowing offensive linemen to block with arms fully extended. In 1985, this was taken a step further to allow this type of blocking in all situations. Mair's group believes that this blocking technique, with arms fully extended and elbows "locked," places the athlete at increased risk for posterior labral injury.[31] All 9 athletes in this study were found at surgery to have labral detachments but no evidence of instability. With a posteriorly directed force, the result is a shearing injury to the posterior labrum and articular surface. Labral reattachment provided good results in all of these athletes.

Linemen are also at increased risk of these posterior shearing forces because of the importance placed on bench pressing. This type of strength training drives the humerus posteriorly across the posterior labrum.

True posterior instability (and recurrent posterior instability) is much less common than anterior instability, and isolated posterior labral detachments or tears. However, because of the mechanisms described earlier, it is much more common in football players. Recognition of this entity on MR imaging is critical when treating these athletes. Findings that may be seen include posterior capsular lesions, humeral avulsion of the posterior inferior glenohumeral ligament (PIGHL), intrasubstance ligament attenuation, and combined lesions.

Disruption of both the humeral and glenoid attachments of the anterior inferior glenohumeral has been described previously.[35] This condition has been termed the "floating anterior inferior glenohumeral ligament lesion," indicating complete detachment at both attachments. More recently, humeral and glenoid avulsion of the posterior band of the inferior glenohumeral ligament has been described.[5,36–39]

Recurrent posterior instability resulting from a posterior Bankart lesion, associated with a posterior humeral avulsion of the inferior glenohumeral ligament, has been described. This combination of abnormality is referred to as a *floating PIGHL* lesion. The authors have seen this lesion in several football players, both at the collegiate and professional level (**Figs. 4 and 5**).[36,40]

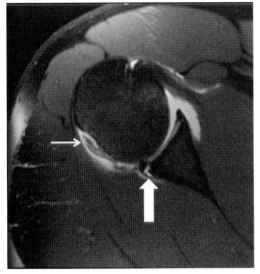

Fig. 4. "Floating posterior inferior glenohumeral ligament" lesion in an NFL offensive lineman. Axial T_1-weighted fat-saturated MR arthrographic image shows contrast within the base of the posterior labrum and periosteum (*thick arrow*), indicating detachment, and an avulsed, retracted posterior capsule/inferior glenohumeral ligament (*thin arrow*).

Slap Tears

Snyder was the first to introduce the term *SLAP* lesion while defining an injury to the superior glenoid labrum that "begins posteriorly and extends anteriorly" (superior labrum anterior-posterior).[40,41] This injury may be acute or chronic, and their causes are well documented in the throwing athlete. They are thought to be a result of traction across the long head of the bicep during the deceleration phase of throwing.[42] Additional causes may include internal impingement[43] and the "peel-back mechanism" secondary to a posterior

dominant biceps attachment.[44] However, Funks' group looked at 18 contact sport athletes (rugby players) and found that all of the SLAP tears were related to a direct lateral blow to the shoulder during a heavy tackle.[44] Snyder's group observed 140 SLAP tears in nonathletes and found this cause in 31% of patients.[45]

The typical clinical presentation was that of a painful clunking in the shoulder. Maximum pain occurred during bench pressing, and most often was felt during descending the weights (eccentric connection), and not at the end range of the lifts (differentiating from acromioclavicular joint abnormality).[46]

MR and MR arthrography are the preferred imaging modalities in detecting SLAP tears.[47–52] Four types of SLAP tears are commonly described, although further classification has described up to 12 variants. Type I is irregularity of the labral margin with mild increased signal intensity, type II demonstrates abnormal signal between the superior labrum and glenoid margin (**Fig. 6**), type III is a bucket handle–type tear involving only the labrum (**Fig. 7**), and type IV is a bucket-type tear that involves the biceps tendon.[18]

Biceps Tendon

The biceps tendon has 2 distinct segments about the shoulder. The first portion is intra-articular and the second dives into the intertubercular groove of the proximal humerus. This second portion is surrounded by a synovial sheath. Tendinosis, subluxation/dislocation, and proximal rupture can all occur to the tendon at the shoulder.

Although ultrasound can occasionally be useful for detecting focal tendon abnormalities, MR imaging is extremely helpful because it can visualize the entire course of the proximal tendon down to the proximal humeral shaft.

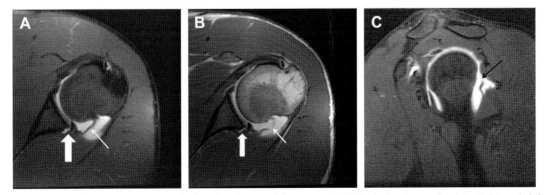

Fig. 5. Partial "floating posterior inferior glenohumeral ligament (PIGHL)" lesion in a collegiate tight end. (*A*) Axial T_1-weighted fat-suppressed MR arthrographic image reveals contrast imbibition within the torn posterior labrum (*thick arrow*), with an intact posterior inferior glenohumeral ligament inferiorly (*thin arrow*), (*B, C*) but torn PIGHL slightly cephalad (*thin arrow*).

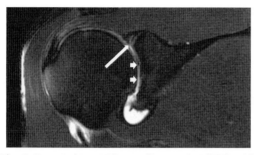

Fig. 6. Type II slap tear in a college quarterback with moderate degenerative changes of the glenohumeral joint space. Coronal oblique T$_2$-weighted fat-saturated MR image shows an incomplete tear of the superior labrum (*long arrow*) with loss of articular cartilage and joint space narrowing (*short arrow*).

Tendinosis is difficult to differentiate from medial subluxation clinically, because both present with pain to the proximal aspect of the groove. MR imaging is important for differentiating these entities, because tendinosis is treated conservatively and medial subluxation/dislocation is treated surgically. In the case of biceps tendon subluxation or dislocation, the transverse bicipital ligament is torn, as are fibers of the distal, cephalad portion of the subscapularis and the remainder of the structures of the biceps sling, including the distal aspects of the coracohumeral and superior glenohumeral ligaments. In contact athletes, surgical intervention is even more critical in returning the athlete to play.[3]

Biceps dislocation occurs most often in football players when a quarterback is hit while throwing. Tension is placed on the biceps tendon with the arm externally rotated, resulting in stripping of the transverse ligament from the lesser tuberosity. This process leads to medial dislocation of the tendon. MR imaging will directly visualize the dislocated tendon (**Fig. 8**). When the tendon reduces with internal rotation of the shoulder, MR imaging can demonstrate associated transverse humeral ligament stripping, allowing accurate diagnosis. Treatment ranges from reconstruction of the transverse humeral ligament and deepening of the groove to biceps release and tenodesis. Although tenodesis is most commonly performed, a loss of function as a humeral head depressor results.[1]

Acromioclavicular Joint

Acromioclavicular separation is the second most common shoulder injury (after traction injury to the brachial plexus ["stingers"]), based on data from college players arriving to the NFL.[53] The mechanism is a fall directly on the point of the shoulder with the arm adducted, depressing the acromion. When the clavicle does not fracture, force is absorbed by the acromioclavicular ligament first, followed by the coracoclavicular ligaments, and finally the deltoid and trapezius muscles, which may partially or completely tear (**Fig. 9**).[1,11] Less commonly, the force is indirect, with a fall on an abducted and flexed arm. Type I injury is a sprain of the acromioclavicular ligament, with point tenderness at the joint, normal radiographs, and edema within the ligament on T$_2$-weighted MR imaging images. Type II injury is disruption of the acromioclavicular ligament and joint capsule on MR imaging, with intact coracoclavicular ligaments, and type III injury is disruption of the coracoclavicular ligaments. In severe injuries, the articular disc may be extruded.

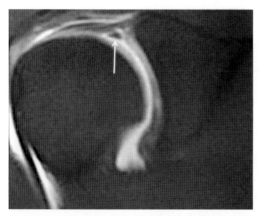

Fig. 7. Type III slap tear. Coronal oblique T$_1$-weighted fat-suppressed MR arthrographic image shows contrast completely surrounding a detached superior labrum (*arrow*), with the adjacent biceps tendon intact.

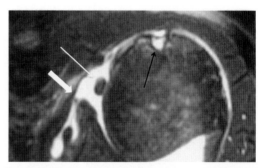

Fig. 8. Medial dislocation of the biceps tendon with complete rupture of the distal subscapularis tendon. Axial T$_2$-weighted fat-suppressed image shows medial dislocation of the biceps tendon into the anterior aspect of the glenohumeral joint space (*long arrow*) with rupture and retraction of the distal subscapularis tendon (*thick arrow*). Note empty bicipital groove (*black arrow*).

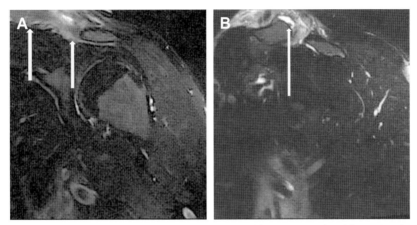

Fig. 9. Trapezius muscle strain and partial avulsion. (*A*) Coronal oblique T_2-weighted fast spin echo image shows diffuse abnormal increased signal within the trapezius muscle belly (*arrow*) and (*B*) partial avulsion of the clavicular origin, with a fluid-filled gap (*arrow*).

Treatment includes modification of shoulder pads with an acromioclavicular doughnut. Even quarterbacks with grade III injuries can respond to nonoperative treatment and return to play within 5 to 6 weeks.[1,11]

ELBOW EPIDEMIOLOGY

Carlisle and colleagues[53] looked at frequency of injuries to the arm, including the elbow, forearm, and wrist, in NFL players over a 10-year period. They found that most of these athletes experienced elbow injuries (58%), with 30% of injuries involving the wrist and 12% involving the forearm. Ligamentous abnormalities were the most common diagnosis in the elbow and wrist, whereas wrist sprains were the most common overall diagnosis. Fractures were the most common injury in the forearm. Forearm injuries led to the most playing time lost (mean of 42 days), most likely because the predominant forearm injury was fracture. Elbow injuries led to an average of only 22 days lost.

Tackling was the mechanism most frequently attributed to causing elbow, wrist, and forearm injuries (24%). Linemen experienced these injuries more commonly than other positions, and elbow injuries were the most common in these players, encompassing 75% of injuries. Defensive backs experienced the most frequent forearm injuries; double that of any other position, probably related to attempting "arm" tackles on high velocity running backs and wide receivers.[54]

Ligament Injury

In contradistinction to the chronic valgus stress seen in overhead throwing athletes, ulnar collateral ligament sprains in football are usually the result of acute trauma. The most common mechanism is direct valgus load applied to the arm while the hand is planted on the surface of the playing field or while blocking at the line of scrimmage. The opposing lineman tries to break free by delivering a blow to the arm leading to the valgus force. The authors saw a high school football player who experienced a ulnar collateral ligament tear with fracture of the radial head from simultaneous forces (helmets) applied to both the radial and ulnar sides of the elbow while the hand was planted on the ground, supporting his body weight (**Fig. 10**). Although ulnar collateral ligament injuries

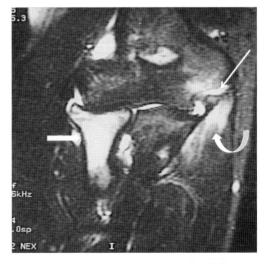

Fig. 10. A 14-year-old high school football player struck on elbow by helmets while hand was planted on ground. Coronal T_2-weighted fast spin echo image shows prominent proximal radius contusion (*thick arrow*), medial condylar avulsion (*thin arrow*) and proximal common flexor muscle strain (*curved arrow*).

can occur as a result of overuse in quarterbacks, this is much less commonly seen in football players than baseball players.

Injury to the lateral ligamentous structures is a well-described entity that often leads to chronic posterolateral rotator instability (PLRI). However, previous reports describe that only 2.9% of elbow injuries in the NFL were related to lateral ligamentous strains.[55] Once these ligaments are disrupted, PLRI symptoms may include clicking, locking, weakness, and functional disability.[56] When symptomatic, most authors advocate reconstructive surgery of the lateral ulnar collateral ligament.[57] The main indications for lateral ligamentous reconstruction of the elbow are elbow dislocation and iatrogenic surgical release.[57] Muller and colleagues[55] reported a case of a 25-year-old wide receiver in the NFL who experienced a contact injury from a valgus force to the elbow, resulting in complete disruption of the radial collateral and lateral ulnar collateral ligaments off of the lateral epicondyle of the humerus. Instead of surgical repair of the lateral ulnar collateral ligament, the athlete was treated conservatively and was able to return to sport without sequelae of his injury.

Elbow Dislocation

In the authors' practice, the most common indication for MR imaging of the elbow in the acutely injured college or professional player is for the evaluation of elbow dislocation. Similar to the mechanism of the acutely injured ulnar collateral ligament, elbow dislocations are believed to occur through a similar mechanism. The player, usually a lineman, has his upper extremity fixed and extended against his opponent. The opponent tries to break free by striking the extended arm. Alternatively, the player, often at a skill position such as quarterback or running back, may be thrown to the ground during a tackle and attempt to brace the fall with an extended arm. Regardless of the precipitating event, the result is levering of the humerus anteriorly with the elbow in the locked, fully extended position.

The elbow is composed of 3 separate articulations: the ulnotrochlear, radiocapitellar, and proximal radioulnar joints. What these articulations allow for with respect to mobility, they give up in stability, making the elbow the second most commonly dislocated large joint in adults.[58] Adolescent men are at the highest risk for dislocation, and 35% to 75% of all acute elbow dislocations occur in relation to sports activities. The highest-risk sport pertaining to dislocation in women is gymnastics, and in men it is football (representing 22% of all sports-related elbow dislocations).[59–61]

Most simple elbow dislocations, defined as a primary soft tissue injury without associated fractures of the humerus, radius, or ulna, do not usually necessitate operative treatment.[58,62]

MR imaging is critical for the assessment of football players with acute elbow dislocations. In these athletes, injury can occur to virtually all of the primary restraints, and MR imaging plays an important role in determining what additional osseous and soft tissues may be involved. In the acutely dislocated elbow, the anterior and posterior capsules are nearly always disrupted. This abnormality is best seen on sagittal images (**Fig. 11**). The radial, ulnar, and lateral ulnar collateral ligaments are nearly always disrupted. The common flexor and common extensor tendons may be involved. The cubital tunnel retinaculum may be stripped from the medial epicondyle, allowing superficial displacement of the ulnar nerve (**Fig. 12**). Variable partial-thickness tearing of the brachialis muscle is a well-known entity associated with these injuries, with the authors noting it as a constant finding in athletes with this injury (**Figs. 13** and **14**). However, perhaps the most important role of MR imaging in these injuries is the ability to detect fractures, and possibly displaced fractures with loose intra-articular bodies, because this may potentially convert a nonoperative case into an operative one.

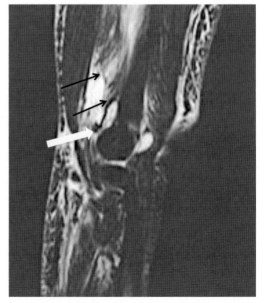

Fig. 11. Acute elbow dislocation with anterior capsular rupture. Sagittal T$_2$-weighted fast spin echo image reveals complete avulsion of anterior joint capsule (*thick arrow*) and high-grade brachialis strain (*black arrows*).

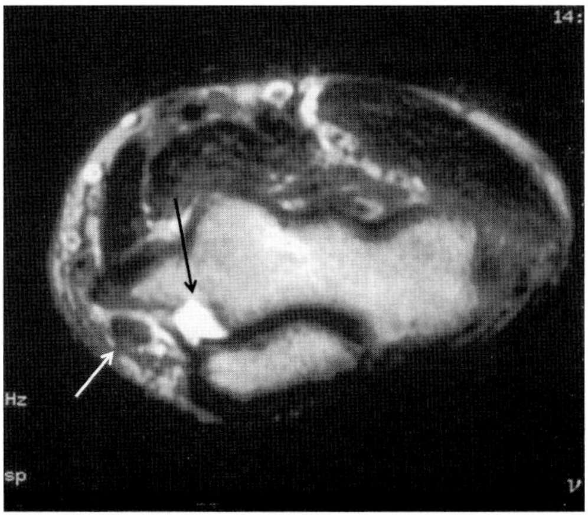

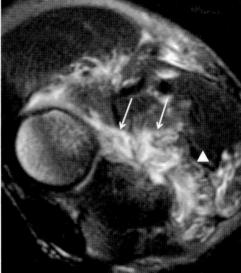

Fig. 12. NFL lineman with elbow dislocation and medial dislocation of the ulnar nerve. Axial T_2-weighted fast spin echo image shows edematous dislocated ulnar nerve (*white arrow*) with an empty cubital tunnel (*black arrow*).

TENDON INJURIES
Triceps Ruptures

Triceps tendons injuries are a rare occurrence. The most comprehensive study examining the football population was performed by Mair and colleagues,[32] who examined 19 professional football players. Most were linemen and the average age was 29 years. Ten partial- and 11 full-thickness tears were identified in these athletes (2 players experienced bilateral injuries). The partial tears were, for the most part, treated conservatively and healed well. All of the full-thickness tears were

Fig. 14. NFL defensive back with acute elbow dislocation while making a one-handed tackle. Axial T_2-weighted fast spin echo image shows high-grade brachialis strain (*arrows*) and common flexor strain (*arrowhead*).

treated surgically and the players were able to return to play by the following season.[63]

Five of the patients had antecedent corticosteroid injections into the olecranon bursa; none claimed anabolic steroid use.[63]

MR imaging is important in these athletes for diagnosing, localizing, and determining extent of injury, because treatment method depends on the findings. In addition, MR imaging showed

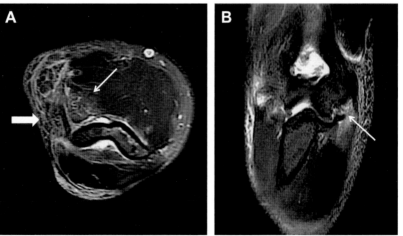

Fig. 13. Offensive lineman with acute elbow dislocation. (*A*) Axial T_2-weighted fast spin echo image reveals abnormal increased T_2 signal intensity (*thick arrow*) within the common flexor muscle group and medial aspect of brachialis (*thin arrow*). (*B*) Complete rupture of the ulnar collateral ligament (*arrow*).

that the partial tears often had a predilection for the medial portion of the tendon in these players.[63]

OSTEOCHONDRAL ABNORMALITIES AND LOOSE BODIES

Although osteochondral abnormalities and injuries have been described extensively in the adult, pediatric, and adolescent thrower, osteochondral injury will also occur in the contact athlete. Injury to the articular surface of the distal humerus may affect the capitellum or trochlea.[64] When present, injury to the capitellum may represent an actual osseous fracture or a manifestation of a dormant osteochondritis dissecans lesion. Hamilton described the case of a 28-year-old professional offensive lineman with symptoms of catching and locking while extending his arm to block.[64] He had an osteochondritis dissecans–type capitellar fracture, which was excised. In football linemen, axial loading force across the radial head to the capitellum is the most likely mechanism, with the degree of elbow flexion or extension at the time of injury determining whether the fracture fragment is displaced anteriorly or posteriorly. Changes from the old blocking rules to allow linemen to engage the defensive player with extended elbows facilitates loading of the capitellum, and this type of injury.[65]

Whether related to previous elbow fractures, repetitive microtrauma, or instability, football players experience degenerative joint disease. Associated chondral loss, osteophytes, and loose bodies will be present. Imaging, whether with plain radiographs, computed tomography (CT), or MR, is critical in determining the degree of joint destruction and the presence of intra-articular loose bodies (**Figs. 15** and **16**).

PECTORALIS MAJOR MUSCLE/TENDON TEARS

The pectoralis major muscle is a triangular-shaped muscle with origins from the clavicle, sternum, ribs, and external oblique fascia. The muscle fibers coalesce into 3 separate laminae that twist 90° before fusing into a single sheet-like tendon that is 5 cm wide and 5 mm thick. Thus, the lowest fibers of the muscle insert the highest on the crest of the greater tuberosity of the humerus.[3,65] This anatomy results in maximum tension on the inferior portion of the muscle tendon unit.[66] The major function of the pectoralis major includes adduction, forward elevation, and inward rotation of the upper extremity.

The pectoralis can tear from direct or (more commonly) indirect trauma. Typically, the musculotendinous junction or tendon ruptures from an eccentric overload, whereas the muscle is maximally contracted. In a football player, this occurs most often while blocking an opponent or during weightlifting, specifically during bench press. The short inferior fibers of the sternal head are the most common site of rupture because of the greater tension placed on them.[3,65–68]

The player often reports an audible "pop" or "snap" with immediate pain. Prominent ecchymosis is usually present in the acute setting along the chest wall and upper arm.[3] Ecchymosis is usually absent in pectoralis minor injuries.[69] Deformity is usually present, and can manifest as either an enlarged axillary fold in a proximal muscle injury

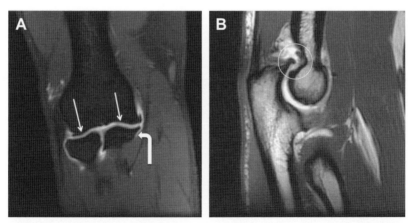

Fig. 15. Collegiate defensive lineman with severe degenerative joint disease of the elbow. (*A*) Coronal T_1-weighted fast spin echo MR arthrographic image of the elbow shows marked narrowing of the radiocapitellar and ulnotrochlear joints (*thin arrows*). Note arthrographic "T" sign, indicative of a partial-thickness chronic ulnar collateral ligament tear (*curved arrow*). (*B*) Sagittal T_1-weighted MR arthrographic image shows osteophytosis of the posterior ulnotrochlear joint.

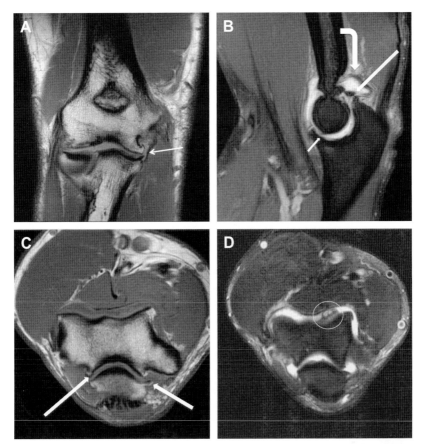

Fig. 16. A 31-year-old veteran NFL offensive lineman with chronic elbow pain and stiffness. (A) Coronal proton density (PD)–weighted image shows prominent medial osteophytosis (*arrow*). (B) Sagittal T_2-weighted fast spin echo image reveals narrowing of the ulnotrochlear compartment (*short arrow*) with a loose body posteriorly (*long arrow*). Thickening of the posterior capsule (synovitis) is present (*curved arrow*). (C) Axial PD-weighted image shows medial and lateral osteophytes (*arrows*), with a loose body also present (D) in the anterior recess (*circle*).

or a chest wall bulge in a distal injury. Associated weakness in adduction and occasionally inward rotation and forward elevation are present. The injury is classified by degree and location. The tear can be partial or complete, with partial injuries being more common. Injury can occur at the muscle origin, muscle belly, musculotendinous junction, or tendinous insertion. Prognosis depends on location and degree of tear. Muscle or musculotendinous injuries are usually partial, treated conservatively, and heal well. Tendinous or tendon insertion tears less than 50% thickness are usually treated conservatively. High-grade partial- or full-thickness tears/avulsions are treated surgically (Fig. 17).

An accurate diagnosis in these athletes is essential to ensure a positive result. MR imaging has proven critical in assessing these injuries. Carrino and colleagues found MR accurate and useful in detecting and grading tears involving

the pectoralis major muscle and tendon, identifying the complete tears that necessitated surgical repair.[67] The authors' institution predominantly uses axial T_1- and T_2-weighted fast-spin echo (FSE), sagittal T_1- and T_2-weighted FSE, and coronal T_1 and short tau inversion recovery (STIR) pulse sequences. Oblique coronal STIR and oblique sagittal T_2 FSE pulse sequences parallel and perpendicular to the long axis of the pectoralis tendon are added in assessment of these athletes (Fig. 18).

PECTORALIS MINOR TEARS

The pectoralis minor muscle is a triangular muscle located deep in the pectoralis major and originates from the second to the fifth ribs and the overlying fascia. It passes superiorly and laterally to insert on the coracoid process of the scapula. The muscle protracts and depresses the lateral angle

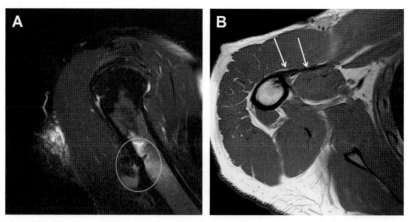

Fig. 17. NFL tight end with pain while bench pressing during off-season workouts 2 years after pectoralis major rupture and surgical repair. (A) Sagittal T_2-weighted fast spin echo image shows postoperative changes within the proximal humeral diaphysis and mild marrow edema (circle). (B) Axial T_1-weighted image shows a normal postoperative pectoralis major tendon, without evidence of re-tear (arrows).

of the scapula. Zvijac and colleagues[68] described 2 cases, one a national football league fullback and the other a lineman, who experienced isolated tears of the pectoralis minor muscles diagnosed with MR imaging. The mechanism of injury was blocking with the shoulder in flexion and the arms extended. Physical examination differed from pectoralis major tears in that no deformity or ecchymosis was present. MR imaging revealed abnormal signal in the region of the coracoid process of the scapula with distinct rupture of the tendon. The patients were treated conservatively and healed well.

COSTOCHONDRAL INJURIES

Identification of the causes of anterior chest wall pain may be a diagnostic dilemma in the elite athletic population. Costochondral injuries must be included, along with rib fractures, sternoclavicular injuries, and pectoralis major and minor tears, among the diagnostic considerations for anterior medial shoulder pain and anterior arm pain.[66,70–72]

These injuries typically occur in young patients as a result of significant trauma, often associated with contact sports. Typically these are seen in wrestlers and hockey and football players.[73,74] The injuries often involve costochondral separation, frequently at the first and second ribs and the sternochondral and costochondral junctions.[75,76] The injuries, as in the case of wrestlers, may be from twisting force to a relatively immobile ribcage, as opposed to injury to the lower ribs, which are the result of a direct blow to the chest.

Radiographs, although helpful for detecting osseous fractures, are insensitive for detecting

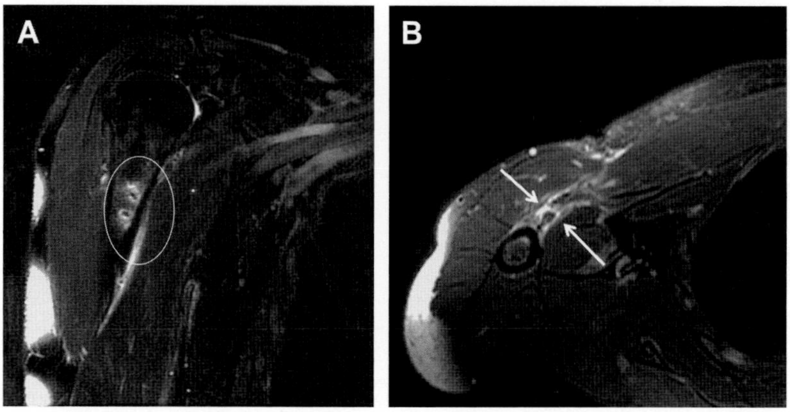

Fig. 18. A 28-year-old NFL offensive lineman with re-tear of pectoralis major tendon while blocking. (A) Oblique coronal STIR image shows susceptibility artifact related to suture anchors. (B) Axial T_2-weighted FSE image reveals complete rupture of the pectoralis major tendon repair (arrows).

cartilage and soft tissue abnormalities.[77] CT, sonography, and MR imaging are more sensitive for detecting these areas.[72] Malghem and colleagues[72] described a series of 8 patients with 15 costal cartilage injuries diagnosed on CT (all 8 patients) and sonography (3 patients).

Subhas and colleagues showed that costochondral injuries are easily seen on MR imaging.[72] Fluid-sensitive pulse sequences revealed high-signal edema in the soft tissues, with resolution of this signal abnormality on routine follow-up MR imaging. The investigators believed that cost-ochondral abnormalities were more conspicuous on MR imaging than on CT, and recommend MR imaging with at least 1 fat-saturated T_2 weighted or STIR sequence in the coronal view when evaluating these patients.[70]

The authors' practice has seen several college and professional football players with pure chondral fractures of the ribcage. In addition to the fluid-sensitive and STIR pulse sequences, the authors have added gradient-echo pulse sequences in the axial plane, and an oblique coronal plane oriented to the symptomatic region. These gradient-echo sequences delineate the costochondral junction and directly visualize the chondral fractures, with or without displacement (Fig. 19). Because of the poor visualization of costal cartilage, they do not use CT in these instances.

WRIST AND HAND INJURIES

Injuries to the distal forearm, carpus, and hand are frequently seen in patients engaged in contact sports. In the youth football player, injuries to the wrist and hand account for approximately 10% of all injuries, second only to the knee.[78,79] Most

are contusions and sprains. Fall on an out-stretched hand results in a compressive force through the carpus into the distal radioulnar joint, which can cause trauma to the osseous structures (fracture) or soft tissues (ligament/cartilage). Football players will frequently ignore these injuries initially, leading to difficult delayed diagnoses and subsequent sequelae, such as osteoarthritis (Fig. 20).

Osseous structures of the wrist include the distal radius and ulna, and the carpus. The distal radius is commonly fractured, and the injury can be intra- or extra-articular. If nondisplaced, these fractures require immobilization in a below-elbow cast for 6 weeks. The athlete may be allowed to return to play during this time. If the fracture is displaced, a reduction will usually be required, and if displaced greater than 2 mm, open reduction and internal fixation are necessary. While casted, the player may return to play, depending on position (ie, nonquarterbacks and nondominant-hand running backs and wide receivers). Radiographs alone are adequate for evaluating most distal radial fractures. Occasionally, intra-articular fractures will need to be evaluated with additional imaging, such as CT or MR, for assessment of articular offset, alignment, or other associated soft tissue abnormalities.

Scaphoid fractures are the most common carpal fracture, constituting more than 60% of all carpal injuries. They are most common in young men and can be seen in 3 distinct locations: the tuberosity, the waist, and the proximal pole. Waist fractures are the most common and account for 70% of all scaphoid fractures.[18,80,81] A scaphoid fracture should be suspected in any player with wrist pain and tenderness at the anatomic snuffbox. Swelling or ecchymosis is usually absent on

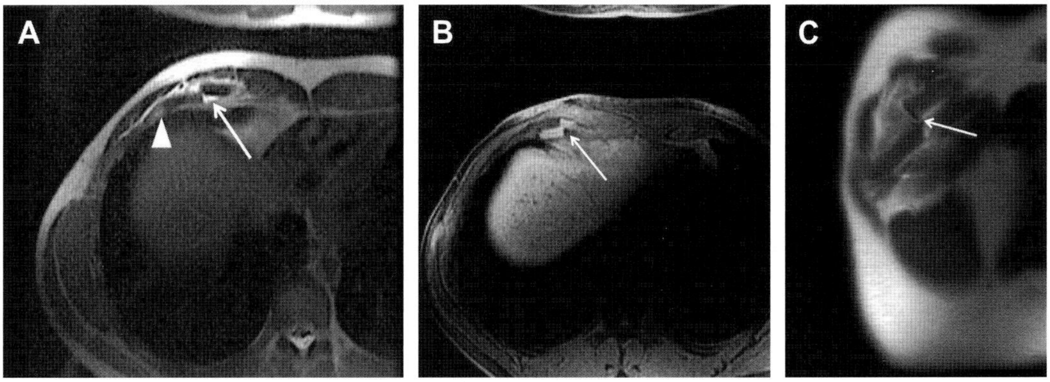

Fig. 19. NFL running back complaining of severe chest and arm pain after being tackled, showing a fracture of costal cartilage. (A) Axial T_2-weighted, (B) gradient echo, and (C) oblique coronal T_1 images showing complete fracture of the costal cartilage with overriding of the fracture fragments (arrows). Note the costochondral junction (arrowhead).

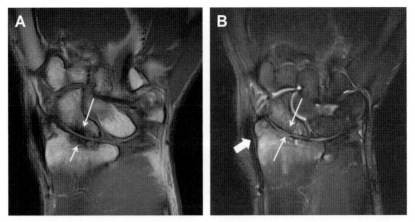

Fig. 20. Collegiate quarterback with osteoarthritis and severe wrist pain and decreased range of motion. (*A*) Coronal proton density (PD)–weighted non–fat-saturated and (*B*) coronal PD-weighted FSE images show marked narrowing of the radioscaphoid joint space with subchondral sclerosis and reactive marrow change (*thin arrows*). Old fracture deformity of the radial styloid is present (*thick arrow*).

physical examination. Initial radiographs are often negative or inconclusive, and these athletes must be treated as if fractured until proven otherwise. MR imaging is often used to make a definitive diagnosis in these individuals because of its ability to reveal a low-signal intensity fracture line, and marrow edema.[81–85] T_1 and STIR imaging in the coronal planes are useful for identifying fracture and edema, whereas sagittal images are best to assess for fracture fragment displacement, such as humpback deformity.

A common complication of scaphoid fractures is avascular necrosis. The blood supply to the scaphoid arises from dorsal and volar branches of the radial artery and enters through the distal half of the bone.[86–88] Thirty percent of fractures involving the middle third of the scaphoid, and up to 100% of fractures of the proximal pole, lead to avascular necrosis of the proximal fragment.[75,89] Plain radiographs have traditionally been used to assess avascular necrosis of the scaphoid. Changes of increased density in the proximal pole fragment have been used to diagnose this entity in the past. Unfortunately, these plain-film findings lag behind onset of the disease and may not be reliable in predicting viability of the proximal pole fragment.[76] MR imaging has proven helpful in the assessment of scaphoid avascular necrosis.[90–94] Findings include decreased T_1 signal intensity within the proximal pole fragment and may be related to fibrosis, sclerosis, or marrow edema.[95] Fluid-sensitive pulse sequences, such as T_2 or STIR, will show low signal intensity when fibrosis/scarring is present. When viability is in question, intravenous gadolinium is administered. If enhancement is present, proximal pole vascularity persists.[92,96–99] At the authors'

institution, gadolinium is used regularly in athletes in whom scaphoid avascular necrosis is a concern.

The distal radioulnar joint is complex in that the distal ulnar articular surface covers two-thirds of its circumference. This surface articulates with the sigmoid notch of the distal radius, allowing pronation and supination of the forearm and hand. The triangular fibrocartilage complex (TFCC) stabilizes the joint intrinsically, whereas the interosseous membrane, extensor carpi ulnaris, and pronator quadrates muscle stabilize the joint extrinsically. Injuries to the TFCC can occur acutely or may be related to chronic repetitive overuse. In the acute setting, injury may result from axial loading across the distal radius. This injury may occur in a fall on an outstretched hand, with force being transmitted through the thenar eminence musculature, resulting in proximal migration of the radius. This process stretches the TFCC over the ulnar head, leading to injury. Sudden pronation or supination may also cause injury. Partial tears or thinning of either the proximal or distal surfaces and radial- or ulnar-sided tears may be seen. Abnormal increased T_2 or STIR signal within the TFCC, and adjacent high T_2 signal fluid within the distal radioulnar joint or radiocarpal joint may be seen on MR imaging. Many elite athletes will not undergo arthrography, and at the authors' institution, MR imaging is routinely performed in these patients.

Degenerative Arthritis

As with other joints in football players, the wrist tends to undergo degenerative osteoarthritis at an early age. This finding is particularly true for the distal radioulnar, radiocarpal, and midcarpal joints of the wrist, because these athletes tend to "play through" the ligamentous and cartilaginous injuries for an extended period before diagnosis. The subsequent altered mechanics lead to cartilage loss and joint space narrowing. The degree of functional loss depends on the severity of the injury and the position of the player. A quarterback who loses mobility in his throwing hand will be much more affected by degenerative changes than the nonquarterback. However, if the changes are pronounced, very few positions will be able to compete without some significant loss of function.

Plain radiographic findings of degenerative changes include subchondral sclerosis, subchondral cystic change, osteophytosis, and joint space narrowing. MR imaging findings include subchondral reactive increased T_2 or STIR signal within the marrow, subchondral low T_1 and T_2 signal representing sclerosis, and joint space narrowing. A high-quality MR imaging study can exquisitely show chondral loss, often early in the degenerative process.

Ligament Injuries of the Wrist and Hand

The main intrinsic ligaments of the wrist are the scapholunate and lunotriquetral ligaments. Athletes frequently ignore and underreport these injuries initially. The altered mechanics of the wrist, and the pain and subsequent degenerative changes, may lead to significant disability and loss of playing time for these athletes. Injury to these ligaments usually results from a single traumatic event. Radiographs are usually nondiagnostic. In the nonathletic population, triple arthrography is often used to diagnose intrinsic ligament tears. In the elite athlete, however, invasive studies such as arthrography are not well tolerated. Therefore, MR imaging is used.

Scapholunate ligament injury presents with pain, swelling, and tenderness over the dorsoradial aspect of the wrist. Tears may be partial or complete, and may involve the dorsal, volar, radial, or ulnar aspects. Discontinuity or complete absence of a portion of the ligament may be seen. MR imaging may show fluid signal within the ligament, more commonly the volar portion, because this is the area of weakest ligamentous attachments.

The lunotriquetral interosseous ligament is smaller than the scapholunate ligament, and therefore tears in these structures are more difficult to detect. Fortunately, these lesions are less common. Lunotriquetral ligament injuries have several causes. Disruption may be related to perilunar instability, a component of ulnocarpal

abutment syndrome, or secondary to a loading force in maximal extension, radial deviation, and possibly pronation.[18] Patients typically present with ulnar-sided pain.

Ulnar collateral ligament injury to the thumb ("gamekeeper's thumb") is a result of a radially directed force on an abducted thumb. This entity was described extensively elsewhere in this issue. In football players, grabbing a ball handler (ie, quarterback, running back, or wide receiver) and having the thumb suddenly jerked in a radial direction while holding onto a jersey may cause this injury (**Fig. 21**).

Tendon injuries typically involve the extensor carpi ulnaris, the first extensor compartment, and the flexor tendons, although any tendon can be involved. Tendinosis and tenosynovitis may be seen as areas of tendon thickening or abnormal increased T_2 or STIR signal intensity on MR imaging. Partial- or full-thickness ruptures may occur as a chronic or acute injury. A partial- or full-thickness defect may be seen with fluid signal intensity on water-sensitive MR pulse sequences. Magic angle phenomenon may be seen in the tendons of the wrist, particularly along the extensor tendons, and particularly the extensor pollicis longus tendon as it traverses the Lister tubercle and

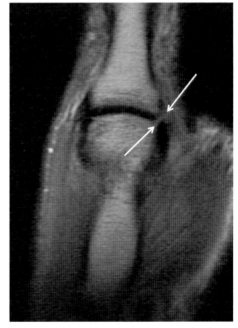

Fig. 21. Professional football player with distal tear of the ulnar collateral ligament at the metacarpophalangeal joint of the thumb. Coronal proton density–weighted MR image of the thumb shows complete tear of the distal ulnar collateral ligament (*arrow*). No Stener lesion is present.

heads to the thumb metacarpal. The possibility of this phenomenon should always be taken into consideration when assessing this region.

SUMMARY

Imaging of football players is unique in many ways. Familiarity with mechanisms of injury, position of the player, and the need for rapid diagnosis and reporting will help radiologists when dealing with these athletes. Although plain radiographs are typically the first imaging modality used, MR imaging has become the cornerstone on which diagnoses and treatment decisions are based. As these athletes become stronger, faster, and more skilled, the ability to accurately assess their injuries becomes even more important, and understanding of the challenges that these patients present becomes critical.

REFERENCES

1. Wasudev NP, Ho CP. Mechanisms and imaging of football-related injuries. Semin Musculoskelet Radiol 2005;9(4):302–15.
2. Metzl JD. Sports-specific concerns in the young athlete: football. Pediatr Emerg Care 1999;15(5): 363–7.
3. Jackson C, Tyer B. Football. In: Pettrone FA, editor. Athletic injuries of the shoulder. New York: McGraw Hill; 1995. p. 343–5.
4. Browne MG, Nicholas SJ. Upper extremity injuries in American football. In: Nicholas JA, Hersaman EB, Posner MA, editors. The upper extremity in sports medicine. 2nd edition. St Louis (MO): Mosby; 1995. p. 863–82.
5. Seto JL, Brewster CE, Shields CL. Shoulder injuries in football. In: Andrews JR, Wilk RE, editors. The athlete's shoulder. New York: Churchill Livingstone; 1994. p. 391–7.
6. Culpepper MI, Niemann KM. High school football injuries in Birmingham, Alabama. South Med J 1983;76(7):873–5, 878.
7. Andresen BL, Hoffman MD, Barton LW. High school football injuries: field conditions and other factors. Wis Med J 1989;88(10):28–31.
8. Kaplan LD, Flanigan DC, Norwig J, et al. Prevalence and variance of shoulder injuries in elite collegiate football players. Am J Sports Med 2005;33(8):1142–6.
9. Neer CS 2nd. Impingement lesions. Clin Orthop Relat Res 1983;(173):70–7.
10. Meister K. Injuries to the shoulder in the throwing athlete. Part two: evaluation/treatment. Am J Sports Med 2000;28(4):587–601.
11. Kelly BT, Barnes RP, Powell JW, et al. Shoulder injuries to quarterbacks in the national football league. Am J Sports Med 2004;32(2):328–31.
12. Fleisig GS, Escamila RF, Andrew JR, et al. Kinematic and kinetic comparison between baseball pitching and football passing. J Appl Biomech 1996;12:207–24.
13. Wick H, Dillman CJ, Werner S. A kinematic comparison between baseball pitching and football passing. Sports Med Update 1991;6:13–6.
14. Blevins FT, Hayes WM, Warren RF. Rotator cuff injury in contact athletes. Am J Sports Med 1996;24(3):263–7.
15. Gorse KM, Myers JB, Radelet M, et al. An acute, traumatic supraspinatus lesion in an intercollegiate football player: a case report. J Athl Train 2000; 35(2):198–203.
16. Iannotti JP, Zlatkin MB, Esterhai JL, et al. Magnetic resonance imaging of the shoulder. Sensitivity, specificity, and predictive value. J Bone Joint Surg Am 1991;73(1):17–29.
17. Fritz RC. Magnetic resonance imaging of sports-related injuries to the shoulder: impingement and rotator cuff. Radiol Clin North Am 2002;40(2):217–34.
18. Edelman R, Crues JV, Zlatkin MB, et al. Shoulder. In: Clinical magnetic resonance imaging, Vol. 3. Philadelphia: Saunders; 2006. p. 3204–79.
19. Rowe CR, Patel D, Southmayd WW. The Bankart procedure: a long-term end-result study. J Bone Joint Surg Am 1978;60(1):1–16.
20. Marans HJ, Angel KR, Schemitsch EH, et al. The fate of traumatic anterior dislocation of the shoulder in children. J Bone Joint Surg Am 1992;74(8):1242–4.
21. Mazzocca AD, Brown FM Jr, Carreira DS, et al. Arthroscopic anterior shoulder stabilization of collision and contact athletes. Am J Sports Med 2005;33(1):52–60.
22. Cho NS, Hwang JC, Rhee YG. Arthroscopic stabilization in anterior shoulder instability: collision athletes versus noncollision athletes. Arthroscopy 2006;22(9):947–53.
23. Hubbell JD, Ahmad S, Bezenoff LS, et al. Comparison of shoulder stabilization using arthroscopic transglenoid sutures versus open capsulolabral repairs: a 5-year minimum follow-up. Am J Sports Med 2004;32(3):650–4.
24. Larrain MV, Montenegro HJ, Mauas DM, et al. Arthroscopic management of traumatic anterior shoulder instability in collision athletes: analysis of 204 cases with a 4- to 9-year follow-up and results with the suture anchor technique. Arthroscopy 2006;22(12):1283–9.
25. Lynch JR, Clinton JM, Dewing CB, et al. Treatment of osseous defects associated with anterior shoulder instability. J Shoulder Elbow Surg 2009;18(2):317–28.
26. Robinson CM, Jenkins PJ, White TO, et al. Primary arthroscopic stabilization for a first-time anterior dislocation of the shoulder. A randomized, double-blind trial. J Bone Joint Surg Am 2008;90(4):708–21.
27. Brophy RH, Gill CS, Lyman S, et al. Effect of shoulder stabilization on career length in national football league athletes. Am J Sports Med 2011; 39(4):704–9.

28. Escobedo EM, Richardson ML, Schulz YB, et al. Increased risk of posterior glenoid labrum tears in football players. AJR Am J Roentgenol 2007; 188(1):193-7.

29. Weinberg J, McFarland EG. Posterior capsular avulsion in a college football player. Am J Sports Med 1999;27(2):235-7.

30. Hawkins RJ, Janda DH. Posterior instability of the glenohumeral joint. A technique of repair. Am J Sports Med 1996;24(3):275-8.

31. Mair SD, Zarzour RH, Speer KP. Posterior labral injury in contact athletes. Am J Sports Med 1998; 26(6):753-8.

32. Antoniou J, Harryman DT 2nd. Posterior instability. Orthop Clin North Am 2001;32(3):463-73.

33. Harryman DT 2nd, Sidles JA, Harris SL, et al. The role of the rotator interval capsule in passive motion and stability of the shoulder. J Bone Joint Surg Am 1992;74(1):53-66.

34. Field LD, Bokor DJ, Savoie FH 3rd. Humeral and glenoid detachment of the anterior inferior glenohumeral ligament: a cause of anterior shoulder instability. J Shoulder Elbow Surg 1997;6(1):6-10.

35. Pokabla C, Hobgood ER, Field LD. Identification and management of "floating" posterior inferior glenohumeral ligament lesions. J Shoulder Elbow Surg 2010;19(2):314-7.

36. Castagna A, Snyder SJ, Conti M, et al. Posterior humeral avulsion of the glenohumeral ligament: a clinical review of 9 cases. Arthroscopy 2007; 23(8):809-15.

37. Chhabra A, Diduch DR, Anderson M. Arthroscopic repair of a posterior humeral avulsion of the inferior glenohumeral ligament (HAGL) lesion. Arthroscopy 2004;20(Suppl 2):73-6.

38. Chung CB, Sorenson S, Dwek JR, et al. Humeral avulsion of the posterior band of the inferior glenohumeral ligament: MR arthrography and clinical correlation in 17 patients. AJR Am J Roentgenol 2004;183(2):355-9.

39. Hill JD, Lovejoy JF Jr, Kelly RA. Combined posterior Bankart lesion and posterior humeral avulsion of the glenohumeral ligaments associated with recurrent posterior shoulder instability. Arthroscopy 2007; 23(3):327.e1-3.

40. Snyder SJ, Karzel RP, Del Pizzo W, et al. SLAP lesions of the shoulder. Arthroscopy 1990;6(4):274-9.

41. Jobe FW, Moynes DR, Tibone JE, et al. An EMG analysis of the shoulder in pitching. A second report. Am J Sports Med 1984;12(3):218-20.

42. Jobe CM. Evidence for a superior glenoid impingement upon the rotator cuff. J Shoulder Elbow Surg 1993;2:519.

43. Burkhart SS, Morgan CD. The peel-back mechanism: its role in producing and extending posterior type II SLAP lesions and its effect on SLAP repair rehabilitation. Arthroscopy 1998;14(6):637-40.

44. Funk L, Snow M. SLAP tears of the glenoid labrum in contact athletes. Clin J Sport Med 2007;17(1):1-4.

45. Snyder SJ, Banas MP, Karzel RP. An analysis of 140 injuries to the superior glenoid labrum. J Shoulder Elbow Surg 1995;4(4):243-8.

46. Beltran J, Jbara M, Maimon R. Shoulder: labrum and bicipital tendon. Top Magn Reson Imaging 2003; 14(1):35-49.

47. Bencardino JT, Beltran J, Rosenberg ZS, et al. Superior labrum anterior-posterior lesions: diagnosis with MR arthrography of the shoulder. Radiology 2000; 214(1):267-71.

48. Waldt S, Burkart A, Lange P, et al. Diagnostic performance of MR arthrography in the assessment of superior labral anteroposterior lesions of the shoulder. AJR Am J Roentgenol 2004;182(5):1271-8.

49. Jee WH, McCauley TR, Katz LD, et al. Superior labral anterior posterior (SLAP) lesions of the glenoid labrum: reliability and accuracy of MR arthrography for diagnosis. Radiology 2001;218(1):127-32.

50. Tung GA, Entzian D, Green A, et al. High-field and low-field MR imaging of superior glenoid labral tears and associated tendon injuries. AJR Am J Roentgenol 2000;174(4):1107-14.

51. Smith AM, McCauley TR, Jokl P. SLAP lesions of the glenoid labrum diagnosed with MR imaging. Skeletal Radiol 1993;22(7):507-10.

52. Schlegel TF, Boublik M, Ho CP, et al. Role of MR imaging in the management of injuries in professional football players. Magn Reson Imaging Clin N Am 1999;7(1):175-90.

53. Carlisle JC, Goldfarb CA, Mall N, et al. Upper extremity injuries in the National Football League: part II: elbow, forearm, and wrist injuries. Am J Sports Med 2008;36(10):1945-52.

54. Kenter K, Behr CT, Warren RF, et al. Acute elbow injuries in the National Football League. J Shoulder Elbow Surg 2000;9(1):1-5.

55. Muller MS, Drakos MC, Feeley B, et al. Nonoperative management of complete lateral elbow ligamentous disruption in an NFL player: a case report. HSS J 2010;6(1):19-25.

56. Mehta JA, Bain GI. Posterolateral rotatory instability of the elbow. J Am Acad Orthop Surg 2004;12(6): 405-15.

57. Kuhn MA, Ross G. Acute elbow dislocations. Orthop Clin North Am 2008;39(2):155-6.

58. Stoneback JW, Owens BD, Sykes J, et al. Incidence of elbow dislocations in the United States population. J Bone Joint Surg Am 2012;94(3):240-5.

59. Josefsson PO, Nilsson BE. Incidence of elbow dislocation. Acta Orthop Scand 1986;57(6):537-8.

60. Linscheid RL, Wheeler DK. Elbow dislocations. JAMA 1965;194(11):1171-6.

61. Cohen MS, Hastings H 2nd. Acute elbow dislocation: evaluation and management. J Am Acad Orthop Surg 1998;6(1):15-23.

62. Mair SD, Isbell WM, Gill TJ, et al. Triceps tendon ruptures in professional football players. Am J Sports Med 2004;32(2):431–4.

63. Rockwood CA, Green DP. Fractures and dislocations of the elbow. Fractures in adults. 2nd edition. Philadelphia: J.B Lippincott Co; 1984. p. 590–5.

64. Hamilton WP, Bennett JB. Capitellum osteochondral injury in a football lineman. Orthopedics 1992;15(6):737–9.

65. Bak K, Cameron EA, Henderson IJ. Rupture of the pectoralis major: a meta-analysis of 112 cases. Knee Surg Sports Traumatol Arthrosc 2000;8(2):113–9.

66. Potter BK, Lehman RA Jr, Doukas WC. Pectoralis major ruptures. Am J Orthop (Belle Mead NJ) 2006;35(4):189–95.

67. Carrino JA, Chandnanni VP, Mitchell DB, et al. Pectoralis major muscle and tendon tears: diagnosis and grading using magnetic resonance imaging. Skeletal Radiol 2000;29(6):305–13.

68. Zvijac JE, Zikria B, Botto-van Bemden A. Isolated tears of pectoralis minor muscle in professional football players: a case series. Am J Orthop (Belle Mead NJ) 2009;38(3):145–7.

69. Ontell FK, Moore EH, Shepard JA, et al. The costal cartilages in health and disease. Radiographics 1997;17(3):571–7.

70. Griffith JF, Rainer TH, Ching AS, et al. Sonography compared with radiography in revealing acute rib fracture. AJR Am J Roentgenol 1999;173(6):1603–9.

71. Miles JW, Barrett GR. Rib fractures in athletes. Sports Med 1991;12(1):66–9.

72. Malghem J, Vande Berg B, Lecouvet F, et al. Costal cartilage fractures as revealed on CT and sonography. AJR Am J Roentgenol 2001;176(2):429–32.

73. Adickes MS, Stuart MJ. Youth football injuries. Sports Med 2004;34(3):201–7.

74. Halpern B, Thompson N, Curl WW, et al. High school football injuries: identifying the risk factors. Am J Sports Med 1987;15(4):316–20.

75. Schmitt R, Heinze A, Fellner F, et al. Imaging and staging of avascular osteonecroses at the wrist and hand. Eur J Radiol 1997;25(2):92–103.

76. Schimmerl-Metz SM, Metz VM, Totterman SM, et al. Radiologic measurement of the scapholunate joint: implications of biologic variation in scapholunate joint morphology. J Hand Surg Am 1999;24(6):1237–44.

77. Kemp SP, Targett SG. Injury to the first rib synchondrosis in a rugby footballer. Br J Sports Med 1999;33(2):131–2.

78. Allan CH, Joshi A, Lichtman DM. Kienbock's disease: diagnosis and treatment. J Am Acad Orthop Surg 2001;9(2):128–36.

79. Cooney WP 3rd. Scaphoid fractures: current treatments and techniques. Instr Course Lect 2003;52:197–208.

80. Brydie A, Raby N. Early MRI in the management of clinical scaphoid fracture. Br J Radiol 2003;76(905):296–300.

81. Gäbler C, Kukla C, Breitenseher MJ, et al. Diagnosis of occult scaphoid fractures and other wrist injuries. Are repeated clinical examinations and plain radiographs still state of the art? Langenbecks Arch Surg 2001;386(2):150–4.

82. Gäbler C, Kukla C, Breitenseher MJ, et al. MRI of occult scaphoid fractures. J Trauma 1996;41:73–6.

83. Thorpe AP, Murray AD, Smith FW, et al. Clinically suspected scaphoid fracture: a comparison of magnetic resonance imaging and bone scintigraphy. Br J Radiol 1996;69(818):109–13.

84. Gelberman RH, Gross MS. The vascularity of the wrist. Identification of arterial patterns at risk. Clin Orthop Relat Res 1986;(202):40–9.

85. Panagis JS, Gelberman RH, Taleisnik J, et al. The arterial anatomy of the human carpus. Part II: the intraosseous vascularity. J Hand Surg Am 1983;8(4):375–82.

86. Gelberman RH, Menon J. The vascularity of the scaphoid bone. J Hand Surg Am 1980;5(5):508–13.

87. Cooney WP, Linscheid RL, Dobyns JH. Scaphoid fractures. Problems associated with nonunion and avascular necrosis. Orthop Clin North Am 1984;15(2):381–91.

88. Cave EF. The carpus, with reference to the fractured navicular bone. Arch Surg 1940;40:54–76.

89. Trumble TE. Avascular necrosis after scaphoid fracture: a correlation of magnetic resonance imaging and histology. J Hand Surg Am 1990;15(4):557–64.

90. Golimbu CN, Firooznia H, Rafii M. Avascular necrosis of carpal bones. Magn Reson Imaging Clin N Am 1995;3(2):281–303.

91. Cristiani G, Cerofolini E, Squarzina PB, et al. Evaluation of ischaemic necrosis of carpal bones by magnetic resonance imaging. J Hand Surg Br 1990;15(2):249–55.

92. Reinus WR, Conway WF, Totty WG, et al. Carpal avascular necrosis: MR imaging. Radiology 1986;160(3):689–93.

93. Perlik PC, Guilford WB. Magnetic resonance imaging to assess vascularity of scaphoid nonunions. J Hand Surg Am 1991;16(3):479–84.

94. Dawson JS, Martel AL, Davis TR. Scaphoid blood flow and acute fracture healing. A dynamic MRI study with enhancement with gadolinium. J Bone Joint Surg Br 2001;83(6):809–14.

95. Cerezal L, Abascal F, Canga A, et al. Usefulness of gadolinium-enhanced MR imaging in the evaluation of the vascularity of scaphoid nonunions. AJR Am J Roentgenol 2000;174(1):141–9.

96. Munk PL, Lee MJ. Gadolinium-enhanced MR imaging of scaphoid nonunions. AJR Am J Roentgenol 2000;175(4):1184–5.

97. Munk PL, Lee MJ, Janzen DL, et al. Gadolinium-enhanced dynamic MRI of the fractured carpal scaphoid: preliminary results. Australas Radiol 1998;42(1):10–5.

98. Zlatkin MB, Greenan T. Magnetic resonance imaging of the wrist. Magn Reson Q 1992;8(2):65–96.

99. Zlatkin MB, Chao PC, Osterman AL, et al. Chronic wrist pain: evaluation with high-resolution MR imaging. Radiology 1989;173(3):723–9.

Index

Note: Page numbers of article titles are in **boldface** type.

Radiol Clin N Am 51 (2013) 331–335
http://dx.doi.org/10.1016/S0033-8389(13)00011-0
0033-8389/13/$ – see front matter © 2013 Elsevier Inc. All rights reserved.